3rd Edition

TYPE 2 DIABETES

Your Healthy Living Guide

*Tips, Techniques and
Practical Advice
for Living Well with
Diabetes*

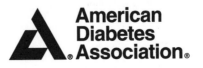

**American
Diabetes
Association®**

Director, Book Publishing: John Fedor
Editor: Janet Cave
Production Manager: Peggy M. Rote
Composition: Circle Graphics
Cover Design: VC Graphics Design Studio
Printer: Transcontinental Printing, Inc.

Printed in Canada
1 3 5 7 9 10 8 6 4 2

The suggestions and information contained in this publication are generally consistent with the *Clinical Practice Recommendations* and other policies of the American Diabetes Association, but they do not represent the policy or position of the Association or any of its boards or committees. Reasonable steps have been taken to ensure the accuracy of the information presented. However, the American Diabetes Association cannot ensure the safety or efficacy of any product or service described in this publication. Individuals are advised to consult a physician or other appropriate health care professional before undertaking any diet or exercise program or taking any medication referred to in this publication. Professionals must use and apply their own professional judgment, experience, and training and should not rely solely on the information contained in this publication before prescribing any diet, exercise, or medication. The American Diabetes Association—its officers, directors, employees, volunteers, and members—assumes no responsibility or liability for personal or other injury, loss, or damage that may result from the suggestions or information in this publication.

∞ The paper in this publication meets the requirements of the ANSI Standard Z39.48-1992 (permanence of paper).

ADA titles may be purchased for business or promotional use or for special sales. For information, please write to Lee Romano Sequeira, Special Sales & Promotions, at the address below.

American Diabetes Association
1701 North Beauregard Street
Alexandria, Virginia 22311

Library of Congress Cataloging-in-Publication Data

Type 2 diabetes : your healthy living guide : tips, techniques, and practical advice for living well with diabetes.—3rd ed.
    p.cm.
    Includes index.
    ISBN 1-58040-060-4 (pbk. : alk. paper)
    1. Non-insulin-dependent diabetes—Popular works. I. Title: Type two diabetes. II. American Diabetes Association

        RC662.18.T975 2000
        616.4'62—dc21   00-064288

CONTENTS

FOREWORD

Type 2 Diabetes: Your Healthy Living Guide, Third Edition has been updated and expanded to provide you with all the latest information you need to live a healthy life with diabetes. It takes you through the basics of what diabetes is to tips on finding the best medical care and making a plan to care for your diabetes. You'll learn about the newest meal-planning tools and medications and what's expected of you and your health care providers in monitoring your health. You'll find out how to steer clear of diabetes complications, fit diabetes into your lifestyle, and navigate your way through the emotional ups and downs of living with diabetes.

Type 2 Diabetes: Your Healthy Living Guide, Third Edition gives you the tools and techniques you'll need to help you meet the challenge of diabetes. No doubt, in meeting the challenge of diabetes, you will improve your diabetes control. Be sure to ask your health care providers for help when you need it, and try your new-found skills every chance you get. Your reward will be your better health, today and tomorrow.

ACKNOWLEDGMENTS

Many thanks to the reviewers of this book:

R. Keith Campbell, MBA, RPh
Washington State University
Pullman, Washington

Alan M. Jacobson, MD
Joslin Diabetes Center
Boston, Massachusetts

Davida Kruger, MSN, RN, C,
  CDE
Henry Ford Health System
Detroit, Michigan

Marvin E. Levin, MD
Washington School of Medicine
Chesterfield, Missouri

Peter A. Lodewick, MD
Diabetes Care Center
Birmingham, Alabama

Joyce Green Pastors, RD, MS,
  CDE
Virginia Center for Diabetes
  Professional Education
Charlottesville, Virginia

David S. Schade, MD
University of New Mexico
  School of Medicine
Albuquerque, New Mexico

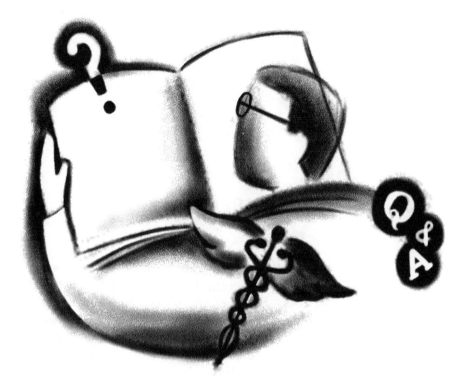

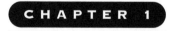

CHAPTER 1

INTRODUCTION TO
TYPE 2 DIABETES

INTRODUCTION TO TYPE 2 DIABETES

WHAT IS DIABETES?

Diabetes is a serious disease that affects your body's ability to change food into energy. Insulin helps you get energy from food. Some of the food you eat turns into a sugar called glucose. Glucose travels around your body in the blood. Your body stores glucose in cells to use for energy. Insulin is the key that opens the door to the cells. In type 2 diabetes, your body does not make enough insulin, or has trouble using the insulin, or both. When you don't have enough insulin or it doesn't work right, the glucose stays in your blood. Over time, glucose will build up in your blood and spill into your urine. This can hurt your eyes, kidneys, nerves, heart, and blood vessels.

Insulin is made by cells in the pancreas called beta cells. When you eat and at other times over the day, the pancreas releases insulin into the blood to take care of rises in glucose. If the beta cells die, insulin is no longer made. This is what happens in people with type 1 diabetes. This is why they must inject insulin to live. A person with type 2 diabetes might inject insulin but does not depend on it to live.

Type 2 diabetes usually comes on slowly. You may have only mild symptoms or not notice any symptoms at all for years. Some common symptoms are constant thirst, constant hunger, frequent urination, blurred vision, and fatigue. You may also experience tingling, numbness, or pain in your hands or feet; dry, itchy skin; and infections of the skin, gums, bladder, or vagina that keep coming back or heal slowly.

WHO GETS TYPE 2 DIABETES?

About 16 million Americans have diabetes. Most of them—9 out of 10—have type 2 diabetes. Type 2 diabetes used to be called adult-onset diabetes. That's because most people who get type 2 diabetes are over 40. But younger people may also get it.

Researchers aren't sure what causes type 2 diabetes. They do know that you can't catch it from someone else, like you can the flu. They know it isn't caused by eating too much sugar. Type 2 diabetes is not a simple disease. You can't pinpoint the one thing that went wrong to cause your diabetes, because it probably wasn't just one thing. It does run in families. If other members of your family have type 2 diabetes, you are more likely to get it. But it usually takes something else to bring on the disease.

For many people, being overweight brings it on. When you are overweight, your body has a harder time using the insulin that it makes. This is called *insulin resistance*. In insulin resistance, your pancreas keeps making more and more insulin to lower blood glucose, but your body does not respond to the insulin as it should. After years of this, your pancreas may just burn out.

Another unhealthy aspect of being overweight is where you are overweight. If you carry most of the extra weight above the belt, you are more at risk for diabetes, high blood pressure, and heart disease.

Many people don't get enough exercise. They may also eat too many foods that are high in fat and sugars and too few foods that are high in starches and fiber. This way of life—high in calories and low in exercise—is probably the main reason that type 2 diabetes is so common.

Women who get a temporary type of diabetes when they are pregnant, called *gestational diabetes*, are more likely to have type 2 diabetes when they get older. Also, women who have had a baby weighing 9 pounds or more are at greater risk for developing type 2 diabetes.

Hispanic, African American, and Native American people are more likely to develop type 2 diabetes, too. Scientists suspect one reason may be that the "thrifty" genes that helped their ancestors survive in periods of famine cause problems now when they eat too much food and get too little exercise.

Are You Overweight?

One way to determine whether you are overweight is to compare your weight to this chart of acceptable weights for men and women.

Height Without Shoes (feet and inches)	Weight Without Clothes (pounds)	Height Without Shoes (feet and inches)	Weight Without Clothes (pounds)
4'10"	91–119	5'9"	129–169
4'11"	94–124	5'10"	132–174
5'0"	97–128	5'11"	136–179
5'1"	101–132	6'0"	140–184
5'2"	104–137	6'1"	144–189
5'3"	107–141	6'2"	148–195
5'4"	111–146	6'3"	152–200
5'5"	114–150	6'4"	156–205
5'6"	118–155	6'5"	160–211
5'7"	121–160	6'6"	164–216
5'8"	125–164		

From the United States Department of Agriculture: *Report of the Dietary Guidelines Advisory Committee on the Dietary Guidelines for Americans*, 1995, p. 10.

What's Your Body Mass Index?

Another way to determine whether you are overweight is to figure out your body mass index, or BMI. To figure out your BMI, multiply your weight in pounds by 705. Divide this answer by your height in inches. Now divide by your height again. The answer is your BMI. Some BMIs are already figured out in the table below.

BODY MASS INDEX (BMI)

Height (inches)	19	20	21	22	23	24	25	26	27	28	29	30	35	40
							Body Weight (pounds)							
58	91	96	100	105	110	115	119	124	129	134	138	143	167	191
59	94	99	104	109	114	119	124	128	133	138	143	148	173	198
60	97	102	107	112	118	123	128	133	138	143	148	153	179	204
61	100	106	111	116	122	127	132	137	143	148	153	158	185	211
62	104	109	115	120	126	131	136	142	147	153	158	164	191	218
63	107	113	118	124	130	135	141	146	152	158	163	169	197	225
64	110	116	122	128	134	140	145	151	157	163	169	174	204	232
65	114	120	126	132	138	144	150	156	162	168	171	180	210	240
66	118	124	130	136	142	148	155	161	167	173	179	186	215	247
67	121	127	134	140	146	153	159	166	172	178	185	191	223	255
68	125	131	138	144	151	158	164	171	177	184	190	197	230	262
69	128	135	142	149	155	162	169	176	182	189	196	203	236	270
70	132	139	146	153	160	167	174	181	188	195	202	207	243	278
71	136	143	150	157	165	172	179	186	193	200	208	215	250	286
72	140	147	154	162	169	177	184	191	199	206	213	221	258	294
73	144	151	159	166	174	182	189	197	204	212	219	227	265	302
74	148	155	163	171	179	186	194	202	210	218	225	233	272	311
75	152	160	168	176	184	192	200	208	216	224	232	240	279	319
76	156	164	172	180	189	197	205	213	221	230	238	246	287	328

Find your height in the left column. Move across the row to find your weight. The number at the top of the column is your BMI.

To find out whether you are overweight, compare your BMI to the figures below:

▪ A BMI of 20 to 25 is normal weight.
▪ A BMI of 25 to 30 is overweight.
▪ A BMI of 30 or greater is severely overweight.

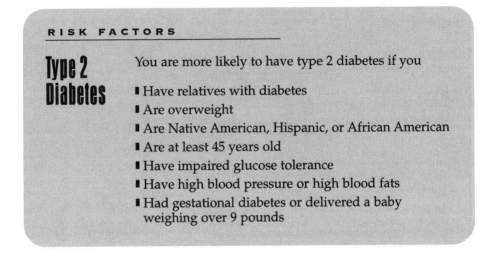

RISK FACTORS

Type 2 Diabetes

You are more likely to have type 2 diabetes if you

- Have relatives with diabetes
- Are overweight
- Are Native American, Hispanic, or African American
- Are at least 45 years old
- Have impaired glucose tolerance
- Have high blood pressure or high blood fats
- Had gestational diabetes or delivered a baby weighing over 9 pounds

WHAT CAN YOU DO ABOUT TYPE 2 DIABETES?

There is no cure for diabetes. Your health care provider cannot give you anything to make it go away. It is a chronic disease. But there are things you can do to treat it yourself. Healthy eating and exercise are the best treatments for type 2 diabetes. Everyone who has diabetes finds it is easier to control if they eat healthy meals and exercise daily.

Certain foods raise your blood glucose. How much a food raises your blood glucose is based on the type of food, how it is prepared, how much you eat of it, when you eat it, and what you eat along with it. You can find out how the foods you eat affect your blood glucose level by testing your blood glucose after eating.

Exercise lowers your blood glucose level by using some of the glucose in your blood. It also helps your muscles use insulin better, so even more glucose is removed from the blood. When you add exercise, such as a 20-minute walk, to your daily schedule, you may lose weight, too. Losing as little as 10 pounds can help some people get their blood glucose levels back to normal.

If healthy eating and exercise do not bring your blood glucose levels down to where you want them, you may need diabetes pills. Diabetes pills are drugs that lower blood glucose levels. They are not insulin. If healthy food, exercise, and diabetes pills do not lower your blood glucose, you may need to take insulin, too. Or you may need to use insulin instead of diabetes pills.

To find out how your treatments are working, there are two things you can do: 1) self-monitor your blood glucose levels, and 2) have regular medical checkups. With a blood ·glucose meter, you can check your blood glucose level at any time of the day and see what effect the food you ate, or the exercise you did, had on your blood glucose level. This helps you make decisions—what to eat, when to exercise, or how much medication to take—to control your blood glucose level. This knowledge can give you more flexibility in your day-to-day activities, too. When you can predict what your blood glucose level will do, you can change your schedule around—eat at a later time, exercise more than usual—and still keep your blood glucose levels under control.

By using a blood glucose meter, you don't have to wait until you go to your health care provider to know how you are doing. Still, your health care provider is important. Only your health care provider can check your overall health to assess how your treatments are working. Having a physical exam at least once a year gives your health care provider a better chance of finding any potential problems.

WHY DOES DIABETES CONTROL MAKE SENSE?

Untreated type 2 diabetes can lead to serious diseases of the heart, blood vessels, nerves, kidneys, and eyes. These diseases are called diabetes complications. You may have had diabetes for years and not even known about it. During that time, high blood glucose levels may have been damaging these parts of your body. That is why it is important for you to take control of diabetes as soon as you are diagnosed.

You can do something to prevent or postpone diabetes complications. Bringing your blood glucose levels closer to normal will stop or slow the damage to your eyes, nerves, and kidneys. This has been confirmed by two different studies—the 1998 United Kingdom Prospective Diabetes Study (UKPDS) and a 10-year study called the Diabetes Control and Complications Trial (DCCT) The DCCT is the best-known research done on the connection between blood glucose levels and complications. Most

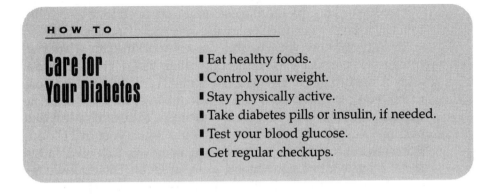

HOW TO

Care for Your Diabetes

▮ Eat healthy foods.
▮ Control your weight.
▮ Stay physically active.
▮ Take diabetes pills or insulin, if needed.
▮ Test your blood glucose.
▮ Get regular checkups.

of the people who lowered their blood glucose levels benefited. Although the DCCT followed people with type 1 diabetes, the UKPDS showed that people with type 2 diabetes seem to get the same benefits of fewer complications when they reach better blood glucose control. More research is being done in this area.

HOW CAN YOU PROTECT YOUR FAMILY FROM TYPE 2 DIABETES?

Because you have diabetes, your children, siblings, or parents may be at risk for developing it, too. There are ways to help protect them:

- Share your healthy eating plan with your family. Prepare family meals that everyone can enjoy.
- Involve your family in your education. Encourage them to visit your diabetes care provider, dietitian, and other health care team members with you.
- Make sure your family members have regular checkups with a health care provider experienced in diabetes. There are tests that can detect markers for diabetes before it develops.
- Ask your family members to be your exercise partners. Set goals together, and help keep each other motivated.

Developing and maintaining good eating and exercise habits can mean the difference between life with type 2 diabetes and life without it.

HOW DO YOU LIVE WITH DIABETES?

At first, you'll need some time to absorb all the information your health care providers give you. You may feel overwhelmed by all you must do and remember. You may feel sad about the loss of your good health. You may feel angry because you have to make changes to the way you live. You may feel afraid of having a low blood glucose reaction, having to give yourself shots, or the thought of future complications. These and other strong emotions are all part of living with a chronic disease.

Knowing these emotions are part of the disease may help you recognize them more quickly when they appear. This may help you accept your anger, your fear, or your resentment. Seeking support from your family, friends, or a mental health professional may help.

Hopefully, you will come to accept your diabetes. Just realize that even after you have accepted it, you won't always want to follow a healthy meal plan and exercise. Some days will be easier than others. But that's okay. Just do the best you can at the moment, and start fresh each day.

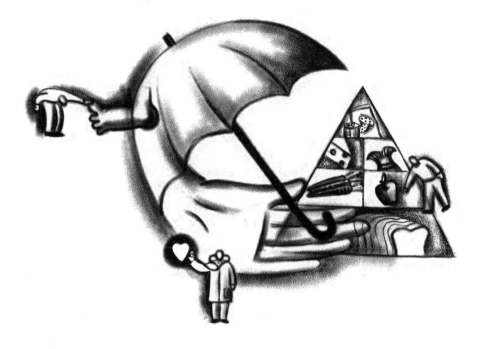

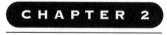
CHAPTER 2

FINDING THE BEST CARE

FINDING THE BEST CARE

Finding the best possible health care is important. At some point, you may need to look for various health care providers, such as a dietitian, an eye doctor, or a foot doctor. Once in a while, you may want to take diabetes education classes. Some day, you may need care at a hospital or a nursing facility or from a home health care agency. Always, you'll need health insurance to help pay for this care.

YOUR DIABETES CARE PROVIDER

Look for a health care provider with experience in diabetes. You may choose an internist, a family practitioner, a general practitioner, a nurse practitioner, or a physician's assistant who cares for people with diabetes. You may also be able to choose an endocrinologist or a diabetologist. An endocrinologist is a medical doctor who has special training and certification in treating diseases such as diabetes. A diabetologist is a medical doctor who has a special interest in diabetes.

If you are looking for a diabetes care provider, you might check with friends or relatives who have diabetes and are satisfied with their medical care, get referrals from health care providers you know and trust, or try a referral service sponsored by your local hospital or a professional medical society (see RESOURCES).

If possible, schedule an appointment just to talk with the provider. Some providers charge for this time, so be sure to ask whether there will be an "interview" fee. During the interview, take time to look over the office. Is the staff polite? How long are you kept waiting past your appointment time? Are educational materials on display?

When interviewing the diabetes care provider, you may want to ask questions such as these:

- How many of your patients have diabetes?
- Do you treat more people with type 1 or with type 2 diabetes? How many patients with type 2 diabetes do you see a month?
- Do you know about the American Diabetes Association (ADA) Standards of Medical Care for People With Diabetes?
- Will the care you give me follow those standards?
- How often will regular visits be scheduled? How often will you check my feet and my glycated hemoglobin, or HbA_{1c}? (The HbA_{1c} test will give you and your doctor a measurement of your day-to-day diabetes control over a 3–4 month period.)
- Who covers for you on your days off?
- What do I do in an emergency?
- Are you associated with other health care providers so that I can benefit from a team approach?

Evaluating your interview is just as important as asking the right questions during it. This is the way to find a competent diabetes care provider with whom you are comfortable. Consider the following questions:

- How do you feel about the interview?
- Did the provider seem genuinely concerned about you?
- Did the provider seem experienced with diabetic patients?
- Did you feel free to speak up?
- Was the provider listening?
- Were the questions you asked answered to your satisfaction?

- Did the provider seem understanding?
- Will you be comfortable working with this provider?

Communication doesn't always come easily. This can be especially true when you're feeling nervous, worried, or under pressure. Here are some tips for smooth communication between you and your diabetes care provider:

- Before your visit, write down what you want to say to your diabetes care provider so you don't forget anything while you're there.
- Ask specific questions, if you can. Your diabetes care provider will answer your questions best if he or she clearly understands what you are asking. For example, if you've been constipated since you started taking a drug, instead of asking "Does this drug cause any side effects?" ask "Does this drug cause constipation?"
- If your diabetes care provider uses words that are too technical and you don't understand what is being said, ask for an explanation.
- Ask your diabetes care provider to repeat anything you didn't hear. Take the time to write down information or instructions.
- Remind your diabetes care provider of previous decisions, lab results, or symptoms. It's not fair to expect the provider to remember everything about you from visit to visit.
- If your diabetes care provider gives advice that you know you can't or won't follow, for whatever reason, say so. Try to work out a different plan.
- Consider bringing a support person (spouse or relative) to sit in on the visit. Sometimes, a second pair of ears will hear things a bit differently.

YOUR HEALTH CARE TEAM

Once you've chosen your diabetes care provider, ask him or her to help you put together a health care team. A health care team is a group of health care providers who help you manage your diabetes. Your team can help you make diabetes care a part of your life.

You are the most important member of the health care team. Only you can do the exercising, follow the meal plan, take the medication, and monitor the results. You'll be the first to notice any problems. You're also likely to be the first to take action. All team members will rely on you to tell them how your diabetes care plan is working and when you need their help.

Your health care team may include, at one time or another, your diabetes care provider, a nurse, a dietitian, a mental health professional, an exercise physiologist, an eye doctor, a foot doctor, a dentist, a pharmacist, and other specialists as needed.

Your diabetes care provider may already use a team approach. If not, ask if he or she would be willing to try such an approach. If your diabetes care provider agrees, ask for referrals to a dietitian, a nurse, or other medical specialists whose help you need.

When selecting members for your health care team, consider asking these questions:

- How many of your patients have diabetes?
- Do you see more people with type 1 or with type 2 diabetes? How many people with type 2 diabetes do you see a month?
- Are you willing and able to work with my diabetes care provider and other team members?
- Will you send regular reports to my diabetes care provider?
- What are the costs of your services? Are they covered by my insurance plan?

Once you have assembled your team, give each team member the name, phone number, fax number, and address of the others to put in your file in their offices. Ask your health care team members to consult each other on your care when appropriate. It's particularly good to do this when specific issues arise or when changes in your diabetes care plan are being considered. For example, let each team member know if you are starting a weight-loss diet, taking an aerobics class, or starting a new medication.

If you have limited access to health care providers, perhaps because of where you live or the type of health insurance you have, see how much of a health care team you can build. Then take responsibility yourself, if necessary, for communicating your test results and treatments from one provder to another.

You may have to do some reading to keep informed on advances in diabetes care.

Dietitian

A dietitian is an expert in food and nutrition. Food is a key part of your diabetes care. A dietitian can help you figure out your food needs based on your weight, lifestyle, diabetes pills or insulin, other drugs you may be taking, and your health goals. Dietitians can teach you many useful skills, such as how to

- Make a meal plan.
- Use a meal plan.
- Fit favorite foods into your meal plan.
- Make a sick-day meal plan.
- Read food labels.
- Choose wisely when grocery shopping.
- Choose wisely from restaurant menus.
- Turn a fatty recipe into a low-fat one.
- Find cookbooks and food guides.
- Find out how the foods you eat affect your blood fat levels.
- Find out how the foods you eat affect your blood glucose levels.
- Test your blood glucose with a glucose meter.
- Treat yourself for low blood glucose.
- Use your blood glucose records to improve your food choices.

When your weight, lifestyle, or health goals change, your food needs will change, too. Your dietitian can help you adjust your meal plan to those changes. Perhaps you just don't like your meal plan. Maybe it needs to fit your daily schedule better. A dietitian can help you do this.

Look for the initials RD after a dietitian's name. RD stands for registered dietitian. A registered dietitian has met standards set by The American Dietetic Association. An RD may also have a master's degree.

You might see the initials LD after a dietitian's name. LD stands for licensed dietitian. Many states require dietitians to have a license.

Your diabetes care provider or local hospitals may be able to recommend a dietitian. Or The American Dietetic Association Consumer Nutrition Hot Line, at 1–800–366–1655, can refer you to a dietitian.

Nurse

Look for the initials RN after a nurse's name. RN stands for registered nurse (RN). Some nurses also have a bachelor's degree (BSN) or a master's degree (MSN). Nurses teach and advise you on the day-to-day management of your diabetes. Nurses can teach you what diabetes is and how to

- Use diabetes pills.
- Use insulin.
- Give yourself insulin shots.
- Use an insulin pump.
- Test your blood glucose.
- Keep track of your diabetes control.
- Know the signs of low and high blood glucose.
- Take care of low or high blood glucose.
- Handle sick days.
- Stay healthy during pregnancy.

Exercise Physiologist

An exercise physiologist is trained in the science of exercise and body conditioning. An exercise physiologist helps you plan a safe, effective exercise program. Look for someone with a master's or doctoral degree in exercise physiology. Or find a licensed health care provider who has graduate training in exercise physiology. Certification from the American College of Sports Medicine is a good sign.

Exercise physiologists can plan individual exercise programs tailored to your specific needs. Perhaps you want to improve your cardiovascular fitness, lower your blood glucose, lose some weight, or develop muscle tone and flexibility. An exercise physiologist can show you the safest exercises for you, whether you have arthritis, are overweight, have complications of diabetes, or have been sitting for years and now want to become more active. Always get your diabetes care provider's approval on any exercise program.

Mental Health Professional

Mental health professionals include social workers, psychologists, and psychiatrists. All are trained to help you with the emotional side of diabetes management. Since diabetes can be a stressful disease, this kind of help is commonly recommended.

Look for a licensed clinical social worker (LCSW) with a master's degree in social work (MSW) and training in individual, group, and family therapy. Social workers can help you and your family cope with any stress or anxieties related to diabetes. They can help you locate community or government resources to help with medical or financial needs.

A clinical psychologist has a master's or doctoral degree in psychology and training in individual, group, and family psychotherapy. Clinical psychologists counsel patients with emotional problems.

A psychiatrist is a medical doctor who can provide counseling for emotional problems and the stresses of diabetes, and prescribe drugs to treat these problems.

Dentist

At first it may seem odd to think of your dentist as a member of your health care team. But dentists have the important role of helping you maintain a healthy mouth and strong teeth. Having diabetes puts you at risk for gum disease and other mouth infections. It's important to have a dental checkup every 6 months and to tell your dentist that you have diabetes.

Eye Doctor

Your eye doctor is either an ophthalmologist or an optometrist. Ophthalmologists are doctors who detect and treat eye diseases. They may prescribe eye medicines and perform eye surgery. Optometrists are not medical doctors. They are trained to examine the eye for vision problems and other minor problems.

Your eye doctor will monitor any changes in your eyes, determine what those changes mean, and discuss with you how best to treat your eyes. The ADA recommends that you have yearly dilated eye and visual exams.

Foot Doctor

A foot doctor is called a podiatrist. A podiatrist is trained to treat foot and lower-leg problems. Podiatrists have a doctor of podiatric medicine (DPM) degree from a college of podiatry. They have also done a residency (hospital training) in podiatry. Foot care is especially important, because people with diabetes are highly likely to get foot problems. Minor foot problems can turn into serious foot problems quickly.

The ADA recommends that you have your feet examined at every regular visit to your diabetes care provider. If you or your diabetes care provider finds any problems with your feet or lower legs, you may want to see a podiatrist. To find a podiatrist, check with your diabetes care provider, area hospitals, or your local ADA affiliate or chapter (see RESOURCES).

Pharmacist

A pharmacist is trained in the chemistry of drugs and how drugs affect the body. A pharmacist has at least a bachelor of science in pharmacy degree (BScPharm) or a doctor of pharmacy degree (PharmD). Your pharmacist can help you in several ways. Most pharmacists offer free counseling. They can tell you

- How often to take your prescription drugs.
- Whether to take your drugs with meals or on an empty stomach.
- What side effects to watch for.
- Whether to stay out of the sun.
- What foods to avoid.
- What other drugs might react with your new drug.
- When to take a missed dose.
- How to store your drugs.
- What nonprescription drugs work best with your other drugs.

Certified Diabetes Educator

The letters CDE after a person's name stand for certified diabetes educator. When you see these letters, you know the person is specially trained to teach or care for people with diabetes. These letters may come after the names of any of the people on your health care team.

A diabetes educator becomes certified by passing a test offered by the National Certification Board for Diabetes Educators—an independent organization established by the American Association of Diabetes Educators. The test covers medications, monitoring, biological changes and complications, psychological issues, and education principles related to diabetes. Once certified, CDEs must stay up-to-date on diabetes care and treatment in order to pass a recertification test every 5 years.

To find a diabetes educator in your area, call the American Association of Diabetes Educators at 1-800-832-6874.

DIABETES EDUCATION CLASSES

A great way for you to keep up with the latest information and ideas about diabetes care is to attend a diabetes education class. To learn about local classes, contact the ADA affiliate or chapter in your state (see RESOURCES or the white pages of your phone book), or ask your local hospitals, the county or state department of health, or your diabetes care provider. Contact each class sponsor and ask for information so you can compare what they have to offer.

Look for diabetes education classes that meet the National Standards for Diabetes Self-Management Education Programs. Many class sponsors advertise it. Classes that meet these standards have skilled and experienced health professionals as instructors, are designed to suit your needs, and should be conveniently located, easily accessible, and able to offer instruction in the following areas:

- Diabetes overview
- Stress and psychological and social issues
- Family involvement and social support
- Food and nutrition
- Exercise and activity

- Medications
- Complications
- Foot, skin, and dental care
- Behavior modification, goal setting, risk reduction, and problem-solving
- Blood glucose control
- Pregnancy and gestational diabetes
- Use of health care systems and community resources

An additional mark of quality is recognition by the ADA. Diabetes education classes voluntarily apply for recognition. All aspects of the diabetes education class are thoroughly reviewed. Contact your ADA affiliate or chapter or the ADA National Center at 703-549-1500 x2403 to find out which diabetes education classes in your area have achieved recognition.

HOSPITAL STAYS

Take the time now to think about how you will handle hospital stays so that you will get the best possible care. Start by learning something about your local hospitals. To learn about a hospital's general reputation, and its reputation for treating people with diabetes, ask your provider where he or she would send a member of his or her family. Ask friends, neighbors, or relatives what they know about local hospitals. Other resources are your ADA affiliate or chapter or a diabetes support group.

Discuss with your diabetes care provider what steps to take if you need emergency hospitalization, and agree on a hospital to use. Perhaps your diabetes care provider has privileges only at certain area hospitals. Or your managed care plan only uses certain hospitals.

Try to learn these important facts about the hospitals you are considering using:

- Which hospitals accept your health insurance?
- Does the hospital have health care providers with diabetes experience on the staff?
- Is there a diabetes education class in the hospital or affiliated with the hospital?

• What other types of support services are available to people with diabetes?

When You're Facing Surgery

Emergency surgery aside, your first question may be whether the surgery is necessary. If a doctor recommends surgery, ask that doctor, and your diabetes care provider, the following questions:

• What other treatments are there, and which are most used?
• What do those treatments involve?
• Why do you suggest surgery for me?
• What is the success rate of the surgery?
• What does the surgery involve?
• What are the risks of the surgery? What are the side effects? How likely are they to happen?
• What will happen if I do not have the surgery?
• Who will do the surgery? Make sure the surgeon that you choose has done this operation often.
• How long will I be in the hospital?
• Will there be restrictions on my activities after surgery? For how long?
• When can I go back to work?
• Will I need follow-up care, such as repeated blood tests, physical therapy, or skilled nursing care?

What to Pack

When you go to the hospital for an operation, be sure to take

• Your blood glucose meter and test strips.
• Your notebook of blood glucose records.
• All your medications in their original bottles.
• A list of your medications, when you take them, and in what dosages.
• A cheap watch or clock.
• Pajamas and slippers.
• Clothes and shoes.

When to Get a Second Opinion

You may want to get a second opinion when

- A provider recommends surgery, long-term medication, or other treatments that will drastically change your life.
- You have doubts about the recommendation or just want reassurance from another provider.
- Your health insurance company insists on a second opinion before paying full coverage for certain treatments or surgery.

When you are searching for a health care provider to give a second opinion, first ask a health care provider you trust. Try calling the appropriate department of a major medical center or teaching hospital. Ask for the name of a specialist in the field.

- Grooming items.
- A notepad and pencils.
- Phone numbers of your family and friends.
- Insurance information.
- Name and phone number of your diabetes care provider.

When You're in the Hospital

Here are some tips to follow while in the hospital. On admission,

- Tell them you have diabetes.
- Give them a list of all medications you are taking, when you take them, and in what dosages.
- Alert them to medications you are allergic to or that cause severe side effects in you.
- Tell them about other medical conditions you have, such as high blood pressure, kidney damage, or eye problems.
- Tell them about any frequent low blood glucose reactions.
- Tell them about your meal plan and any special diets you're on, such as a low-sodium diet.
- Alert them to any food allergies you have.

For the quickest recovery after surgery, have your blood glucose under good control before the operation.

HOME HEALTH CARE

If you are bedridden with a long illness or housebound for a short time, you may want some of the services provided by home health care agencies. These include nursing care and physical, respiratory, occupational, or speech therapy; chemotherapy; dialysis; nutrition and diet therapy; personal care, such as bathing and dressing; and homemaker care. Home health care agencies may provide blood testing or bring a nurse into your home to administer drugs and other treatments.

Home health care agencies include the Visiting Nurses Association, the Veterans Administration, nonprofit public agencies run by city or county health departments, nonprofit private agencies, and for-profit agencies operated by individuals or by corporations. If you are looking for home health care, ask for help or recommendations from

- Your friends, family, and neighbors.
- Your diabetes care provider.
- Your church or synagogue.
- Your county health department.
- Your Area Agency on Aging.
- Your local ADA affiliate or chapter.
- A local hospital's discharge planner or social worker.
- A local senior citizen center or retirement group.
- United Way or other community service organization.
- The reference librarian at your local library.

Once you get the names of agencies, call or visit them, and consider asking the following questions:

- How soon can services begin?
- Are services available 7 days a week, 24 hours a day if needed?
- Must I sign up for a minimum number of hours?
- Will a detailed care plan be prepared before services begin?

- Can I interview potential nurses or aides before they are assigned? Is there a fee for this?
- Can I request a change in nurse or aide?
- What are the fees for various services?
- Will the agency submit bills directly to my insurance company/Medicare/Medicaid?
- Will I get a copy of these bills?
- How often are bills sent?

NURSING FACILITIES

If full-time care is needed, a nursing facility (otherwise known as a nursing home) is often the best option. Nursing facilities can provide medical care (medication, rehabilitation), personal care (help with eating, bathing, dressing), and residential services (room, food, social activities).

Most nursing facilities are for-profit. There are some non-profit nursing facilities owned by fraternal, religious, or civic groups or by local or state governments.

If you are looking for a nursing facility, consult the same sources you would for home health care (above). Once you have found several nursing facilities, call and ask them to send an information packet. Schedule a visit to those facilities that offer the kind of care you seek. You may want to take along a family member or a friend or two. The more eyes the better.

Be sure to check out
- The grounds and outside of the building
- The lobby and hallways
- The bedrooms and bathrooms
- The kitchen and dining room
- The recreation rooms

Be sure to ask about
- Telephones
- Smoke detectors and fire extinguishers
- Emergency exits and call buttons
- Meals and snacks
- Staff members
- Dental services
- Ambulance services

- Religious services
- Recreational activities
- Social and visiting arrangements
- Parking

HEALTH INSURANCE

Caring for your diabetes can be costly, so finding the best possible health insurance coverage is important. Look for a health insurance plan that meets your health care needs as well as your budget. Health insurance plans vary on what parts of your diabetes care they will help pay for. Before you sign up for a health insurance plan, find the answers to these questions:

- Are visits to my diabetes care provider covered?
- Is there a limit on how many times I can see my diabetes care provider in a year?
- How much will I have to pay per visit?
- How much will the plan pay for each visit?
- How much will the plan pay for a hospital stay?
- Is there a limit on what I pay each year?
- Is there a limit on what the plan pays each year?
- Will I be covered right away, or will I have to wait because I have diabetes (a preexisting condition)? How long will I have to wait?
- Does the plan cover blood glucose meters, strips, insulin, syringes, insulin pumps, and other diabetes supplies? Is there a limit on the number of diabetes supplies I can get each month?
- Does the plan help pay for dietitians, mental health professionals, and specialists? Is there a limit on the number of times I can see these providers in a year?
- Does the plan help pay for diabetes education classes?
- What prescriptions are paid for? Is there a prescription plan to reduce costs? How often can prescriptions be refilled? Is there a co-payment fee for each prescription?
- Is home health care covered? Are there any limitations?

If you already have a health insurance plan, call your benefits manager and find out what diabetes-related items your plan does and does not cover. Ask about each item you use. If your plan covers "durable medical equipment," then it may pay for a blood glucose meter, a fingerstick device, an insulin injector or syringes, and an insulin pump, if prescribed by your diabetes care provider as "medically necessary." If your plan covers prescription medications and/or medical supplies, then it may pay for insulin, lancets, glucose meter strips, ketone test strips, and insulin pump supplies, if you have a prescription for them.

Your diabetes care provider may have to provide a thorough explanation in writing of why each of these items is necessary for you. Keep a copy of this explanation. It serves as your "prescription" for these items.

If you believe that your insurance carrier is not covering things that it is supposed to, contact your state insurance department. Each state has its own laws and regulations governing insurance. Several states have recently passed legislation that improves insurance coverage for people with diabetes.

Group Coverage

If you work, your employer may offer you a group health insurance plan. Group plans are usually open to all employees. Your employer may pay most or all of the cost (premium) for you. For an additional fee, these plans may also cover your spouse and children.

If your employer does not offer health insurance, you may still be able to obtain group health insurance through membership in a professional, trade, or religious association, such as the American Bar Association or B'nai B'rith. Benefits vary widely, so be sure to find out what they are.

If you are self-employed, contact your state department of health or insurance commission to find out if your state offers a small-business purchasing pool or a high-risk insurance pool. The cost of insurance pools varies widely among the states, although most try to keep it affordable by placing limits on the premium. There are also several small-business associations, such as the American Business Association, that offer health insurance to members and their employees.

Individual Coverage

If you are not eligible for any form of group health insurance, try to find an affordable individual health insurance policy. Although it can be difficult, it is a necessity for people with diabetes. See **The Health Insurance Portability and Accountability Act of 1996** on p. 30 for more on individual health insurance policies.

Fee-for-Service Plans

In a fee-for-service plan, you and/or your employer pay a yearly fee to an insurance company. The insurance company then pays for all or part of the cost of your medical care. Usually, the insurance company will start paying after you have paid a small amount of the cost, called a deductible.

Many health care providers expect you to pay the total fee at the time of service. You must then apply to your insurance company to receive your reimbursable expenses. Sometimes, however, the provider or hospital will accept assignment of benefits. This means that they will wait for your insurance company to pay its share and then bill you for the remainder.

The biggest advantage of a fee-for-service plan is that you pick the health care providers you want to go to.

Managed Care Plans

Managed care is a general term for an organized group of health care providers. Managed care plans include health maintenance organizations (HMOs), preferred provider organizations (PPOs), and exclusive provider organizations (EPOs). The biggest advantage of managed care plans is that costs are usually lower for you.

Health Maintenance Organizations (HMOs)

An HMO is an organization that hires or contracts with health care professionals to provide a wide range of medical services to individuals and families. Most of the cost of your medical care is covered by a fee paid by you and/or your employer.

Depending on the type of HMO, you may or may not have to satisfy a deductible and/or pay a co-payment at each visit. Also depending on the type of HMO, you may or may not be covered if you go to a provider who is outside the HMO. Before you sign up, be sure to find out how the HMO works.

Preferred Provider Organizations (PPOs)

A PPO is a list of health care providers. The list is prepared and provided by an insurance company. The providers on the list are "preferred" because they have agreed with an insurer to discount their fees.

The preferred providers are paid by the insurer and by a small co-payment from you when you go to them. You may have to pay a small deductible.

You may choose to go to a provider who does not belong to the PPO, but then you pay more.

Exclusive Provider Organizations (EPOs)

An EPO is like a PPO with an important difference. If you choose to go to a provider who does not belong to the EPO, you pay the total bill.

COBRA

COBRA stands for Consolidated Omnibus Budget Reconciliation Act. This federal law lets some people keep their health insurance coverage for a limited time when they would otherwise lose it. You may need health insurance coverage when you are between jobs, when you go from full-time to part-time status, or when you retire. Your dependents may need health insurance coverage if you die or if you and your spouse separate or divorce.

COBRA allows you and your covered dependents to stay covered under your employer's group health insurance plan. Private companies and state and local government offices are covered. Employers with fewer than 20 employees, the federal government, and churches are not covered.

If you want to stay covered, you must notify your employer in writing within 60 days after the event that will cause you to lose coverage. Coverage begins the day you would have lost health insurance. Coverage may last for up to 18 months after you leave your job. If you are disabled, coverage may last up to 29 months. Your dependents may keep coverage for up to 36 months.

You pay the share of the premium you paid before. You usually must pay your employer's share, too. You often pay a small service fee as well. This is almost always less expensive than purchasing a new short-term policy. When your coverage is over, your employer may allow you to convert to an individual policy. Individual coverage is costly, but this option keeps you insured. For more information on COBRA, call the COBRA Hot Line at 202-219-8776.

The Health Insurance Portability and Accountability Act of 1996

The Health Insurance Portability and Accountability Act of 1996 (effective 1 July 1997) makes it easier for people with diabetes to get and keep their health insurance.

According to the Act, insurers and employers may not make insurance rules that discriminate against workers because of their health. And all workers eligible for a particular health insurance plan must be offered enrollment at the same price.

Insurers who sell individual policies must offer an individual policy without preexisting condition exclusions to anyone who 1) has had continuous coverage in a group plan for the previous 18 months, 2) is not currently eligible for coverage under any group plan, and 3) has used up COBRA coverage (see above).

Another part of the Act helps you keep coverage when you change jobs. If you have had diabetes for more than 6 months and have had continuous coverage in an insurance plan, and then leave your job, you cannot be denied coverage by your new employer because of a preexisting condition. If, however, you have been recently diagnosed, that is, up to 6 months ago, and you change jobs, your new employer may refuse or limit your health insurance coverage for 12 months. This is a one-time only waiting period, and it can be reduced by the number of months you had continuous coverage at your previous job. For example, say you were diagnosed with diabetes while employed and covered by your employer's health insurance plan. Five months after the diagnosis, you change jobs. Your new employer may limit or deny your health insurance coverage for the remainder of the 12-month waiting period, or 7 months.

Medicare

Medicare is a federal health insurance program for people age 65 and older and for people who cannot work because of certain disabilities. It is run by the Health Care Financing Administration of the U.S. Department of Health and Human Services. Social Security Administration offices throughout the United States take applications for Medicare.

There are two parts to Medicare: Part A and Part B. Part A helps to pay bills for medical care provided in hospitals, skilled nursing facilities, hospices (for people who are dying), and homes. Medicare will not pay for custodial care provided in a nursing home or private home when that is the only kind of care needed. Custodial care includes help in walking, getting in and out of bed, bathing, dressing, eating, taking medicines, and other activities of daily living.

Part B helps to pay for health provider's services, ambulance services, diagnostic tests, outpatient hospital services, outpatient physical therapy and speech pathology services, and medical equipment and supplies.

If you use insulin, Medicare will help pay for blood glucose meters, lancets, test strips, and other supplies for the meter. Your health care provider must certify in writing that you need all of these items to manage your diabetes. Make copies of your provider's written statement. Give a copy of it to your pharmacist each time you purchase these supplies so that it can be submitted along with your Medicare claim.

Medicare will not pay for diabetes pills, insulin, syringes, or insulin pumps. Medicare also will not pay for regular eye exams, prescription eyeglasses or contact lenses, or routine foot care, such as nail trimming or removal of corns and calluses.

Medicare will help pay for therapeutic footwear and shoe inserts, laser surgery for retinopathy (an eye disease), cataract surgery, kidney transplants, and dialysis.

Medicare may help pay for diabetes outpatient education if it is done in a hospital and prescribed by a health care provider. Medicare may also help pay for outpatient nutrition counseling services or dietitian services.

Most people covered by Medicare get Part A. You can get Part B by paying a monthly fee. Both parts have deductibles and coinsurance amounts that you pay.

For more information on Medicare, call the Medicare Hot Line at 1-800-638-6833. For a free copy of *Your Medicare Handbook*, call Social Security at 1-800-772-1213 or visit your local Social Security Administration office (address found under the U.S. Government listing in your telephone book).

Medigap

Medigap plans cover some of the charges that Medicare doesn't. Medigap plans are sold by private insurance companies. The federal government has defined 10 standard Medigap plans. Some plans may not be offered in your state. You can buy a Medigap plan to pay for prescription drugs, Medicare deductibles, foreign travel emergencies, preventive care, or other costs.

You cannot be denied Medigap coverage if you apply within 6 months of first applying for Medicare Part B. Prices for the same plan vary with insurance companies. Check prices with several insurance companies before you buy a Medigap plan.

For more information about Medigap, ask for a free copy of the *Guide to Health Insurance for People With Medicare* at any insurance company, or call Social Security at 1-800-772-1213 and ask that it be sent to you.

Medicaid

If your income is very low, you might be able to get Medicaid. Medicaid is a federal and state assistance program. Each state decides what income level it thinks is very low. And each state decides what medical services and supplies to cover. Call your state's Medicaid office to find out whether you qualify and what health costs are covered.

Social Security Disability Insurance

If you lose your job because you are disabled, you may be able to get Social Security Disability Insurance. This insurance covers people younger than age 65 who have worked for pay recently and who are now disabled. Social Security has a list of disabilities. If you have a disability on that list and earn less than $500 a month, you are considered disabled. The disabilities that are listed include diabetes with certain kinds of neuropathy, acidosis, amputation, or retinopathy. For more information, call Social Security on weekdays at 1-800-772-1213.

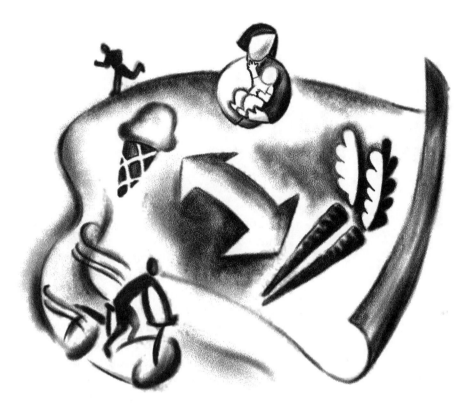

CHAPTER 3

YOUR DIABETES CARE PLAN

YOUR DIABETES CARE PLAN

Taking care of your diabetes is easier if you have a plan. Your diabetes care provider and other members of your health care team can help you make a plan for eating, exercising, weight loss, and medications; a plan for taking care of your eyes, teeth, skin, and feet; even a plan for when you are sick or pregnant.

The goal of a plan is to help you keep your blood glucose level under control and avoid diabetes complications (see Chapter 5). Any plan will need adjusting as you figure out what works best for you and as your needs change.

HEALTHY EATING

Most people with diabetes have an eating plan or meal plan. A meal plan tells you what to eat, how much to eat, and when to eat. A dietitian can help you make a meal plan that is right for you. It should be based on

- What you like to eat and drink.
- When you like to eat and drink.

- How many calories you need.
- The Diabetes Food Pyramid (see below).
- Your level of activity.
- What exercises you do.
- When you exercise.
- Your health.
- What medications you take.
- Your family or cultural customs.

A typical meal plan includes breakfast, lunch, supper, and a bedtime snack. Diabetes meal plans are healthy. Healthy foods for you are the same as for anyone. In fact, your entire family can benefit from the food choices, cooking techniques, and meal-planning tools that you use.

The healthiest eating plan is low in saturated fat and cholesterol, moderate in protein, high in starches and fiber, and moderate in sodium, sugars, and sugar substitutes.

Low in Saturated Fat and Cholesterol

The two main kinds of fat in food are saturated fat and unsaturated fat. Saturated fat is highest in animal foods (meat and dairy products). Cholesterol is found only in animal foods. Saturated fats raise your cholesterol level more than anything else you eat. Most plant foods (fruits, vegetables, grains, legumes, nuts, and seeds) are either low in fat or high in unsaturated fat. Unsaturated fats actually lower your cholesterol level. Most people need only about 30% of their daily calories from fat.

THE HEALTHIEST EATING PLAN		
Low	**Moderate**	**High**
		Starches & Fiber
	Protein	
	Sodium	
Saturated	Sugars	
Fat &	& Sugar	
Cholesterol	Substitutes	

Cooking Tips to Lower Fat and Cholesterol

• Use nonstick cookware, so you won't need to use as much fat.
• Cook food in a tablespoon or less of an unsaturated oil.
• Use nonstick vegetable oil spray, wine, or low-fat or nonfat broth instead of oils.
• Roast, grill, or broil meats on a rack so the fat drains off and away from the food.
• Drain the fat as it cooks out of meats when pan-frying.
• Baste with broth or wine rather than with pan drippings.
• Marinate meats and vegetables in lemon juice, lime juice, sherry, wine, vinegar, low-fat or nonfat broth, or vegetable juice instead of oil. Marinate in herbs and spices, which add flavor with little or no fat or calories.
• Microwave onions, garlic, peppers, and other vegetables in a bit of water instead of sautéing them in oil.
• Skim the fat from soups, stews, broths, gravies, and sauces. Chilling the food in the refrigerator until the fat floats on top and hardens makes the fat easier to remove.

Moderate in Protein

Protein is found in both animal and plant foods. For your good health, it's best to get your protein from foods that are low in fat, calories, and cholesterol.

Good choices for protein are legumes (beans, peas, and lentils), whole grains, and vegetables. All are low in fat and calories and have no cholesterol. Nuts and seeds are also a good choice for protein, because most of the fat they contain is unsaturated.

Meats, poultry, eggs, milk, and cheese are high in protein, but they are also high in saturated fat and cholesterol. If you eat them, stick with lean cuts and low-fat versions. A better choice for protein is fish and shellfish. Most fish and shellfish are lower in saturated fat and cholesterol than meat.

High in Starches and Fiber

Starches are one of the two major types of carbohydrate. The other major type is sugar (discussed below). Carbohydrate is the main nutrient in food that causes your blood glucose to rise. Starches include breads, cereals, pasta, rice, potatoes, corn, whole grains, dry beans, and peas. Most starches have very little fat or cholesterol. Starches that tend to be high in fat, such as biscuits, croissants, muffins, and cornbread, are best avoided.

Fiber, the part of plants that your body can't digest, is part of the total carbohydrate in a food. Fiber is found in fruits, vegetables, whole grains, and legumes (beans, peas, and lentils). All are low in fat and calories and have no cholesterol.

Moderate in Sodium

Many foods contain salt as sodium. Sometimes, you can taste it (as in pickles or bacon). But there is also salt in many foods, such as cheeses, salad dressings, cold cuts, canned soups, and fast foods. The American Diabetes Association (ADA) recommends limiting sodium to no more than 2,400 to 3,000 milligrams a day. Any food with 400 milligrams or more of sodium per serving is considered high in sodium.

Moderate in Sugars

Sugars are one of the two major types of carbohydrate. (The other major type is starches, discussed above.) Carbohydrate is the main nutrient in food that causes your blood glucose to rise. Research has shown that sugars do not raise your blood glucose level any more than starches or other carbohydrates. Because of these findings, a moderate amount of sugars can be part of your healthy eating plan.

Some sugars occur naturally in fruits, vegetables, and dairy products (such as the lactose in milk and yogurt). Foods with natural sugars are usually good sources of vitamins, minerals, fiber, and protein. Sugars may be added to foods during processing. Many nutritious foods, such as breakfast cereals, breads, and low-fat salad dressings, contain some added sugars. Other foods with added sugar, such as chocolate, baked goods, and ice cream treats, give you lots of calories and fat but few nutrients.

Fructose, a sugar found in fruits and vegetables, may cause a smaller rise in your blood glucose level than other sugars. But large amounts of fructose may increase your cholesterol levels.

Because of these findings, there is no reason to use fructose in place of other sugars.

There is also no advantage to using fruit juice or fruit juice concentrates in place of other sugars. They provide the same number of calories, and they raise blood glucose about as high as other sugars do.

Nutrition Facts
Serving Size 1 cup (228g)
Servings Per Container 2

Amount Per Serving

Calories 260   Calories from Fat 120

	% Daily Value*
Total Fat 13g	**20%**
Saturated Fat 5g	**25%**
Cholesterol 30mg	**10%**
Sodium 660mg	**28%**
Total Carbohydrate 31g	**10%**
Dietary Fiber 0g	**0%**
Sugars 5g	
Protein 5g	

Vitamin A 4%	•	Vitamin C 2%
Calcium 15%	•	Iron 4%

* Percent Daily Values are based on a 2,000 calorie diet. Your daily values may be higher or lower depending on your calorie needs:

		Calories:	2,000	2,500
Total Fat	Less than		65g	80g
Sat Fat	Less than		20g	25g
Cholesterol	Less than		300mg	300mg
Sodium	Less than		2,400mg	2,400mg
Total Carbohydrate			300g	375g
Dietary Fiber			25g	30g

Calories per gram:
Fat 9 • Carbohydrate 4 • Protein 4

From U.S. Food and Drug Administration.

Moderate in Sugar Substitutes

Sugar substitutes have very few calories and will not affect your blood glucose level. Unlike sugars, they can be added to your healthy eating plan without taking the place of other carbohydrates. The ADA approves the use of three sugar substitutes in moderate amounts. These are aspartame (Nutrasweet, Equal), saccharin (Sweet'n Low, Sugar Twin, or Sweet 10), and acesulfame potassium (Sweet One or Sunette).

Reading Food Labels

To follow your healthy eating plan, you need to know what nutrients are in the foods you buy. This has been made easier by the fact that most packaged foods now have nutrition labels. The Nutrition Facts label can tell you all you need to know (see Figure).

Nutrition Facts list calories, calories from fat, total fat, saturated fat, cholesterol, sodium, total carbohydrate, fiber, sugars, and protein. Each nutrient is followed by a number. This number is the amount of that nutrient in grams (g) or milligrams (mg) in one serving of the food.

Nutrition Facts also list the amounts of vitamin A, vitamin C, calcium, and iron. Other vitamins and minerals may be listed, too. After the name of the vitamin or mineral is a number followed by a percent sign (%). This number is the percentage of the daily amount of the vitamin or mineral in one serving. Higher numbers mean the food has more of that vitamin or mineral.

Other important numbers on a food label are Daily Values. Daily Values tell you how much total fat, saturated fat, cholesterol, sodium, potassium, total carbohydrate, fiber, and protein you need each day based on the number of calories you eat in a day. There is no Daily Value for sugars.

All Nutrition Facts labels give Daily Values for a person eating 2,000 calories a day, and some labels also give Daily Values for 2,500 calories a day. Your own Daily Values may be higher or lower than those on the label.

The numbers on the right side of the Nutrition Facts label (% Daily Values) tell you what percentage of the Daily Value you are getting in one serving of the food. As a rule of thumb, if the number is 20% or higher, it is enough to be counted in your meal plan. If it is 5% or less, it won't have much effect on your meal plan.

DAILY VALUES FOR 1,200- TO 2,500-CALORIE MEAL PLANS

	Calories Per Day					
Daily Values	**1,200**	**1,500**	**1,800**	**2,000**	**2,200**	**2,500**
Total Fat (g)	40	50	60	67*	73	83*
Saturated Fat (g)	13	17	20	22*	24	28*
Cholesterol (mg)	300	300	300	300	300	300
Sodium (mg)	2,400	2,400	2,400	2,400	2,400	2,400
Potassium (mg)	3,500	3,500	3,500	3,500	3,500	3,500
Total Carbohydrate (g)	180	225	270	300	330	375
Fiber (g)	14	17	21	23*	25	29*
Protein (g)	30	38	45	50	55	63

*These Daily Values appear rounded up or down on food labels.

Serving sizes on food labels are close to what people actually eat, but check before you eat the whole box. One serving may be only half the box, or 3 pieces. If you eat more or less than the serving size, you'll need to adjust the numbers. The serving size is given in both household (e.g., ounces or cups) and metric (e.g., grams) measures. The label also gives the number of servings per container.

Food packages have an ingredients list, too. Ingredients are listed according to their weight in the package. The ingredient weighing the most is listed first. The ingredient listed last weighs the least. It pays to read the ingredients list, because claims on packages can be misleading.

Reading the Nutrition Facts label and the ingredients list on all packaged foods will help you choose the healthiest among them. With a little practice, you'll become familiar with food labels. Then you'll be assured you're getting the nutrients you need and no surprises.

Healthy Choices at the Grocery Store

You'll probably discover that your healthiest food choices at the grocery store don't have food labels. They are vegetables, fruits, legumes, and grains—the foods that come almost directly from the earth to you. Here are some tips on what to look for when buying these and other foods.

Baked goods. Look for baked goods (cakes, cookies, pies, and other desserts) with 3 grams of fat or less per 100 calories.

Breads. Go for breads that list whole grains or multigrains as the first ingredient on the label. Look for those with 2 to 3 grams of fiber, 1 gram of fat or less, and 80 calories per slice.

Canned foods. If you are trying to cut down on salt, choose unsalted canned vegetables and beans. Rinse salted canned foods (vegetables, beans, fish, shellfish, and meats) with cold water for 1 minute to remove some of the salt. Choose unsalted canned tomato sauce, paste, and puree and unsalted broth. Choose canned soups with 400 milligrams or less of sodium and no more than 3 grams of fat per serving.

Cereals. Choose cereals listing whole grains as the first ingredient on the label. Look for breakfast cereals that have

- No more than 2 grams of fat per serving.
- No more than 6 grams of sugars per serving.
- Less than 150 calories per serving.
- Less than 400 milligrams of sodium per serving.
- At least 4 grams of fiber per serving.

Cheeses. Look for skim, low-fat, reduced-fat, or fat-free cheeses. Choose those with 5 to 6 grams of fat or less per 1-ounce serving. Try Alpine Lace cheeses, Kraft Light Naturals cheeses, part-skim and fat-free mozzarella, and farmer cheese. Nonfat or low-fat cottage cheese and ricotta cheese are also good choices.

Cream. Choose nonfat dry milk or condensed skim milk instead of cream or half-and-half. Be wary of powdered nondairy creamers made with palm or coconut oils. They are high in saturated fat. Choose a liquid nondairy creamer made with unsaturated oils.

Fish and shellfish. Choose fresh or frozen fish without batter, breading, or sauces. And select canned fish packed in water without added salt. Or, rinse oil-packed fish under running water to remove some of the added vegetable oil and salt.

Frozen desserts. Look for frozen desserts (yogurt, ice cream, or sherbet) with 3 grams of fat or less and 100 to 150 calories per ½-cup (4-ounce) serving. Frozen low-fat yogurt, fat-free or "light" ice cream, and most sherbets fit in this category. Look for frozen fruit juice bars that have less than 70 calories per bar. Avoid frozen desserts that contain cream of coconut, coconut milk, or coconut oil. These are high in saturated fat.

Frozen dinners. Select frozen dinners that have

- No more than 10 grams of fat per serving.
- Less than 400 calories per serving.
- Less than 50 milligrams of cholesterol per serving.
- Less than 800 milligrams of sodium per serving.

Fruits and fruit juices. Buy fresh, frozen (without added sugar), canned (in water or juice), or dried fruit. If you buy canned fruit packed in syrup, rinse the syrup off under cold water. As for fruit juice, as long as it's 100% (or pure) juice, it can be fresh or from concentrate, canned, bottled, or frozen. Check the label for added sugars and other ingredients you may not want.

Grains. No doubt you've had rice and maybe even brown or wild rice. But there are many other grains to choose from including amaranth, quinoa, buckwheat groats, bulgur wheat, and couscous. And don't forget oats, bran, and wheat germ. Most whole grains contain little fat and 100 calories per ½ cup of cooked grain.

Jams and jellies. Choose fruit spreads, all-fruit jams, or low-sugar spreads. If you eat less than 2 teaspoons per day, they don't count in your calorie total.

Legumes. Legumes include beans, peas, and lentils. Buy dried beans and lentils, fresh or frozen peas, and canned beans without added salt. Choose fat-free varieties of refried beans, baked beans, and vegetarian chili.

Margarine. Choose soft tub, liquid, light, or diet margarine that is labeled low in *trans* fatty acids. *Trans* fatty acids raise low-density lipoprotein (LDL; the bad) cholesterol and lower high-density lipoprotein (HDL; the good) cholesterol. If "partially hydrogenated oil" is listed near the top of the ingredients list, the margarine is high in *trans* fatty acids. Look for a margarine that lists water or liquid vegetable oil as the first ingredient. Buy a margarine that contains no more than 1 gram of saturated fat per tablespoon. Butter contains about 8 grams of saturated fat per tablespoon but no *trans* fatty acids.

Mayonnaise. Look for fat-free or reduced-fat mayonnaise with 5 grams of fat or less per tablespoon.

Meats. Choose lean cuts of meat rather than fatty cuts, and trim off the fat you can see. Wild game, like venison and rabbit, tends to be leaner than other meats.

TOP 5 LEANEST CUTS OF MEATS

Beef	Lamb	Pork	Veal
Top round	Foreshank	Tenderloin	Leg
Eye round	Shank	Sirloin chop	Arm roast
Shank crosscuts	Leg	Loin roast	Sirloin
Tip round	Sirloin	Top loin chop	Blade roast
Bottom round	Arm roast	Loin chop	Loin

Avoid cured or smoked meats, including hot dogs, salami, bologna, bacon, and sausage. These tend to be high in fat. Look for lunch meats with 3 grams of fat or less per ounce.

Milk. Choose skim milk, 1% milk, or buttermilk made from skim milk instead of whole or 2% milk.

Oils. Choose monounsaturated oils, such as olive, avocado, almond, canola, and peanut. And choose polyunsaturated oils, such as corn, safflower, sesame, soybean, and sunflower. Look for oils with no more than 1 gram of saturated fat per tablespoon.

Pasta. Choose fresh or dried pasta. For the least fat, choose pasta made without eggs or oil. Try fiber-rich whole-wheat pasta, low-cholesterol yolk-free pasta, and pasta made with vegetables, such as spinach, tomato, or artichoke.

Poultry. Choose boneless, skinless chicken and turkey breast. They are the leanest. Removing the skin cuts fat and cholesterol. Try ground chicken or turkey in place of ground beef. When buying ground chicken or turkey, check the label for less than 7% to 8% fat by weight (36% or less of calories from fat). Turkey or chicken salami, bologna, hot dogs, and bacon are still high in fat and are best used only occasionally.

Salad dressings. Look for reduced-calorie or fat-free salad dressings with less than 20 to 30 calories and about 5 grams of fat or less per 2 tablespoons. Dilute regular salad dressings with fat-free ones. Or use half a serving (1 tablespoon) of a regular salad dressing. Try flavored vinegars, lemon juice, or just salt and pepper instead of dressing.

Snack foods. Look for crackers, chips, popcorn, and pretzels that are made with whole grains or mostly whole grains. Choose unsalted or lightly salted snacks with 1 to 2 grams of fat per serving.

Soups. Look for canned, dried, or frozen soups with less than 500 milligrams of sodium per 1-cup serving and less than 30% of calories from fat.

Sour cream. Choose light or nonfat sour cream. Better yet, try plain low-fat or nonfat yogurt or pureed low-fat cottage cheese with a little lemon juice.

Vegetables. Choose plain fresh, frozen, or canned vegetables. Avoid vegetables in cream sauces, butter, or margarine.

Yogurt. Choose low-fat or nonfat yogurt instead of whole-milk yogurt. Yogurts sweetened with a sugar substitute are often labeled "lite" and are 50 to 100 calories per serving. Yogurts sweetened with sugar are 150 to 200 calories or more per serving.

Meal-Planning Tools

Now that you have a better idea of what food choices are healthiest, the next step is learning how the food you eat affects your blood glucose level. That's where meal-planning tools come in handy. Three meal-planning tools for people with diabetes are the food pyramid, exchange lists, and carbohydrate counting.

Food Pyramid

For years, the guide to healthy eating had been the Basic Four Food Groups. But in 1992, the U.S. Department of Agriculture (USDA) changed the four food groups into six food groups. And they put the six food groups into sections of a pyramid. They called it the Food Guide Pyramid.

In 1995, The American Dietetic Association and the ADA adapted the USDA Food Guide Pyramid into a pyramid for people with diabetes. It is called the Diabetes Food Pyramid (see below).

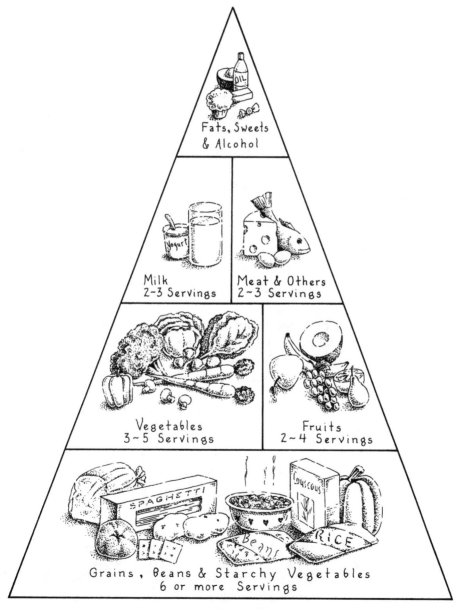

DIABETES FOOD PYRAMID

Your dietitian can help you learn how to divide the recommended number of servings noted on the pyramid into the meals and snacks you eat in a day. When using the pyramid, keep these three things in mind:

Variety. Eat a wide variety of foods from the food groups to get all the nutrients you need. For instance, eat more than one kind of vegetable.

Balance. Eat larger amounts and more servings from food groups that take up more space on the pyramid. The three food groups that take up more space are 1) grains, beans, and starchy vegetables; 2) vegetables; and 3) fruits.

Eat smaller amounts and fewer servings from food groups that take up less space on the pyramid. The three food groups that take up less space are 1) milk; 2) meat and others; and 3) fats, sweets, and alcohol.

Moderation. Eat the right amount of food. How much you eat depends on your health goals, calorie and nutrition needs, activity level, and insulin or diabetes pills. Your dietitian can help you figure out how much to eat.

For more information about using the Diabetes Food Pyramid as a meal-planning tool, see *Diabetes Meal Planning Made Easy: How to Put the Food Pyramid to Work for You, 2nd Ed.*, by Hope Warshaw, MMSc, RD, CDE.

Exchange Lists

Exchange lists are lists of foods grouped together because they are alike. One serving of any of the foods on a list has about the same amount of carbohydrate, protein, fat, and calories. Any food on a list may be "exchanged" or traded for any other food on the same list.

Your dietitian can help you work out a plan using the exchange lists. The meal plan will tell you the number of food exchanges to eat at each meal and snack. You then choose foods that add up to those exchanges.

When choosing foods, be aware that the serving size on a food label may not be the same as the serving size of an exchange. For example, the label may say the serving size of fruit juice is 1 cup, but the exchange list says the serving size of fruit juice is ½ cup. If you drink 1 cup of fruit juice, you need to count 2 Fruit Exchanges, not 1.

With exchange lists, as long as you follow your plan, you are eating a balanced diet. In *Exchange Lists for Meal Planning*, published by the ADA and The American Dietetic Association, there are 15 exchange lists.

CARBOHYDRATES
1. Starch List
2. Fruit List
3. Milk List
4. Other Carbohydrates List
5. Vegetable List

FATS
10. Monounsaturated Fats List
11. Polyunsaturated Fats List
12. Saturated Fats List

MEAT AND MEAT SUBSTITUTES
6. Very-Lean List
7. Lean List
8. Medium-Fat List
9. High-Fat List

OTHER LISTS
13. Free Foods List
14. Combination Foods List
15. Fast Foods List

Carbohydrate Counting

When you eat a healthy meal or snack, it is usually a mixture of carbohydrate, protein, and fat. However, your body changes the carbohydrate into glucose faster than it changes the protein and fat into glucose. It is the carbohydrate that makes your blood glucose level go up. If you know how much carbohydrate you have eaten, you then have some idea how high your blood glucose is going to go.

In carbohydrate counting, you count foods that are mostly carbohydrate. These include starches (breads, cereals, pasta), fruits and fruit juices, milk, yogurt, ice cream, and sugars (honey, syrup). You do not count vegetables, meats, or fats. These foods have very little carbohydrate in them.

You can find out how much carbohydrate a food has by looking at the *Exchange Lists; Carbohydrate Counting Level 1: Getting*

Started; the Nutrition Facts on food labels; and by asking your dietitian.

Knowing how much carbohydrate a food has can help you better control your blood glucose levels. Ask your dietitian or diabetes care provider to help you learn how to use this tool.

EXERCISE

Exercise is as important as food in the treatment of type 2 diabetes. Exercise is good for people with diabetes because it lowers blood glucose levels and often improves the way insulin works in the body.

Types of Exercise

There are three basic types of exercise: aerobic, strength, and flexibility. All three types of exercise work together to make you healthier.

Aerobic exercises are ones that use your heart, lungs, arms, and legs. Aerobic exercises make your insulin work harder and faster, reduce your body fat, and help you lose weight.

Strength exercises are ones that work your muscles against a weight. Strength exercises make your muscles stronger and your bones sturdier. Strong muscles and bones are less likely to become injured.

Flexibility is how far you can stretch your muscles around your joints without stiffness, resistance, or pain. Flexible muscles and joints are less likely to get injured when you use them.

Before You Begin

Before you start any new exercise or exercise program, discuss your plans with your health care team. Your diabetes care provider may want to run some tests to see how your heart, blood vessels, eyes, feet, and nerves are doing. Your blood pressure, blood fat levels, glycohemoglobin levels, and body fat might also be checked.

You and your diabetes care provider may want to work with an exercise physiologist or physical therapist to tailor an exercise program to your needs.

Sample Exercises

AEROBIC EXERCISES
- Aerobics classes or videotapes
- Bicycling
- Dancing
- Jogging
- Jumping rope
- Rowing
- Running
- Skating (roller, ice, in-line)
- Skiing (downhill, cross-country)
- Stair climbing
- Swimming
- Walking
- Water exercises

STRENGTH EXERCISES
- Weight machines
- Free weights
- Calisthenics
- Circuit training

FLEXIBILITY EXERCISES
- Stretching
- Ballet
- Gymnastics
- Martial arts
- Modern dance
- Yoga

Safe Exercising

Some exercises may make any heart, eye, foot, or nerve problems you have worse. Find out from your health care team what kinds of exercises are safe for you to do. From these, pick exercises that will work all your muscle groups (legs and hips, chest, back, shoulders, arms, and abdomen).

Once you have chosen your exercises, learn the right way to do them. If you do exercises the wrong way, you might injure yourself. If the exercises you have chosen require you to use equipment that is new to you, learn how to use and adjust it. Find out how to use any safety equipment that goes along with your exercise, too, such as safety goggles for racquetball and a bicycle helmet for cycling.

Each time you exercise, warm up for 5 to 10 minutes before the exercise, and cool down for 5 to 10 minutes after the exercise. A warm-up will slowly raise your heart rate, warm your muscles, and help prevent injuries. A cooldown will lower your heart rate and slow your breathing. As a warm-up or a cooldown, you could slowly walk or slowly bicycle, then gently stretch.

How Long and How Often to Exercise

If you are just starting to exercise after a long time of little or no activity, go slowly. Doing too much too fast or doing more than you are capable of can lead to injuries that could keep you from doing anything at all.

Start with just 5 minutes of aerobic exercise each day for 1 or 2 weeks. Add 5 more minutes, then another 5. Gradually build up to doing 20 to 60 minutes of continuous aerobic exercise 3 to 5 times a week.

You can even try spreading out your exercise over the day. For example, you might try brisk walking or stair climbing for 10 minutes 2 or 3 times a day or for 15 minutes twice a day. Just be aware that exercising for less than 15 minutes a day is not likely to improve your health.

Start with just 1 set of each strength exercise. (A set is the number of times you repeat an exercise before you rest.) As you become stronger, you will be able to do more sets. Work your way up a little bit at a time to 2 or 3 sets of each exercise. Once you are doing 2 or 3 sets easily, then you are ready to make the exercise harder by adding more weight. Do strength exercises for 20 to 30 minutes 2 or 3 times a week. Allow your muscles at least 1 day of rest between days you do the same strength exercises.

How Hard to Exercise

Your health care provider can tell you how hard to exercise by helping you figure out your target heart-rate range. The following formula is used to calculate target heart rates:

220 − your age = your maximum heart rate in beats per minute.
x 0.60 = your minimum working heart rate in beats per minute.
x 0.80 = your maximum working heart rate in beats per minute.

Activities for the Nonexerciser

If you don't exercise, at least try to be more active. Get on your feet and move around. When you are on your feet and moving around, you are using 2 to 3 times more energy than when you are sitting. Here are some ways to get moving:

▪ Get up to change TV channels instead of using the remote.
▪ Do the ironing while watching TV.
▪ Walk around your house during TV commercials.
▪ Wash dishes, load the dishwasher, or load the clothes washer or dryer during commercials.
▪ Sweep your sidewalk.
▪ Use a rake rather than a leaf blower.
▪ Use a shovel instead of a snow blower.
▪ Use a push lawn mower rather than an electric one.
▪ Plant and maintain an herb or vegetable garden.
▪ Take your pet for a walk.
▪ Play actively with children.
▪ Volunteer to work for a school or hospital.
▪ Walk to the subway or bus stop.
▪ Take the stairs rather than the elevator.
▪ Stand or walk around while you're on the phone.
▪ Walk during lunch, during your break, while the oven is preheating, or while waiting for your prescription.
▪ Run errands that require walking, such as grocery shopping.
▪ Park your car farther away from your destination.
▪ Take a walk with someone you want to talk to.

Using this formula, if you are 55 years old:

$220 - 55 = 165$ beats per minute.
$165 \times 0.60 = 99$ beats per minute.
$165 \times 0.80 = 132$ beats per minute.

This means, your target heart-rate range during exercise is between 99 and 132 beats per minute.

Decide with your health care provider whether to exercise at 60, 70, or 80% of your maximum heart rate. Practice checking your heart rate with your health care team. Then practice at home before trying it while exercising. Here's one way:

• Find your pulse at your wrist or on the front of your neck just below one side of your jawbone. (Caution: Do not check your pulse on both sides of your neck at the same time. You may interrupt blood flow to the brain enough to cause loss of consciousness and possibly a stroke.)
• Watching the second hand of a watch, count the number of heartbeats in 6 seconds, starting with zero.
• Multiply this by 10 to give you the number of beats per minute.

For example, 8 heartbeats x 10 = 80 beats per minute. You can compare this to your working heart-rate range to see whether you are on target.

If you have nerve damage or take certain blood pressure drugs, your heart may beat more slowly. Check with your diabetes care provider about this. If your heart does beat more slowly, your heart rate is not a good guide for how hard to exercise. Instead, exercise at what you feel is a moderate level of exertion. You should be able to talk while you're exercising. And you should not feel that you are working too hard.

SIGNS

You Are Exercising Too Hard

▪ You can't talk while exercising.
▪ Your heart rate is higher than the heart rate you are trying to maintain.
▪ You rate your level of exertion as hard or very hard.

When to Test Your Blood Glucose

Exercise usually makes your blood glucose level go down. But if your blood glucose level is high before you start, exercise can make it go up even higher. It may also go higher if you exercise hard for a short time.

If you take insulin or diabetes pills, exercise can make your blood glucose level go too low. The best way to find out how exercise affects your blood glucose is to test before and after exercising.

Test Your Blood Glucose Twice Before Exercise

Test at 30 minutes before exercise and again just before you begin. This tells you whether your blood glucose level is rising, stable, or dropping. If it is rising, wait until it is stable. If it is dropping, you may need an extra snack to level it off. When it is stable, begin your exercise.

Be Ready to Test Your Blood Glucose During Exercise

There are times during exercise that you may want to stop and check your blood glucose:

- When you are trying an exercise for the first time and want to see how it is affecting your blood glucose
- When you feel your blood glucose might be going too low
- When you will be exercising for more than 1 hour (test every 30 minutes)

Test Your Blood Glucose After Exercise

When you exercise, your body uses glucose that is stored in your muscles and liver. After exercise, your body restores glucose to your muscles and liver by removing it from your blood. This can go on for as long as 10 to 24 hours. During this time, blood glucose levels may fall too low. Watch for this effect during the night or the day after exercising.

When to Eat Snacks

Depending on how hard and how long you exercise, you may need to eat extra snacks. A snack can be a piece of fruit, ½ cup of milk or juice, half a bagel, or a small roll. Talk with your dietitian about what snacks are good for you and when it is best for you to eat them. If you take insulin or diabetes pills, you may need to eat a snack before, during, or after exercise.

If your blood glucose level is less than 100 mg/dl before exercise, you may need to eat a snack before you start. If your blood glucose level is between 100 and 250 mg/dl before exercise and you will be exercising for more than 1 hour, you will need to eat snacks every 30 minutes to 1 hour. If your blood glucose level is between 100 and 250 mg/dl before exercise and you will be exercising for less than 1 hour, you probably will not need to eat a snack.

If you take insulin, you may be able to adjust it instead of eating a snack on the day you exercise. Talk with your diabetes care provider about this.

When and What to Drink

Exercise makes you sweat. Sweating means you are losing fluid. To replace lost fluids, be sure to drink before and after exercise or, if the exercise is intense, during exercise.

Water is usually the best choice. But if you are exercising for a long time, you may want a drink that contains carbohydrate. Choose drinks that are no more than 10% carbohydrate, such as sports drinks or diluted fruit juices (½ cup fruit juice plus ½ cup water).

When to Exercise

A good time to exercise is 1 to 3 hours after you finish a meal or snack. The food you have eaten will help keep your blood glucose level from falling too low.

When Not to Exercise

Do not exercise when

• Your blood glucose level is over 300 mg/dl.

- Your insulin or diabetes pills are at their peak action.
- You have numbness, tingling, or pain in your feet or legs.
- You are dehydrated.
- You are short of breath.
- You are ill.
- You have a serious injury.
- You feel dizzy.
- You feel sick to your stomach.
- You have pain/tightness in your chest, neck, shoulders, or jaw.
- You have blurred sight or blind spots.

How to Stick With It

Convenience. Choose an exercise workout that you can do with a minimum of travel time and preparation. Find something that you can fit easily into your daily routine. Some people find walking at lunchtime convenient. For others, riding a stationary bike at home or taking an exercise class close to home works better.

Cost. Select an activity that requires a minimum of special equipment, clothes, or fees. Consider secondhand exercise equipment. Check out exercise classes at community recreation centers, churches, and schools, where price is usually reasonable.

Classes. Many communities offer a variety of exercise classes. Be cautious, however. Not all exercise classes are equally good. Go watch or try out at least one class before signing up. Look for instructors who are certified and have training in CPR (cardiopulmonary resuscitation). You might also want to ask whether the instructor has experience teaching people with diabetes. Be sure classes include a warm-up, heart-rate monitoring, and a cooldown that includes stretching.

Goals. Set realistic and measurable goals. Work with your health care team on this. Break down the goals, so you can see your achievements. For example, if you're starting a walking program, a short-term goal might be getting out 3 times a week for a month.

Rewards. When you reach a goal, give yourself a reward, such as a new CD, book, or article of clothing.

Enjoyment. Find activities that you enjoy. If you're the social type, chances are you'll enjoy an exercise class. If you value time alone, perhaps swimming laps is for you.

Support. Find someone to exercise with; ask a friend or relative to take a class with you. Making the commitment to meet someone for exercise can help get you out the door.

Learning. Read up on activities you enjoy. Articles, books, or personal accounts of others who enjoy the same activity can be inspirational.

Novelty. If you're bored with the same old exercise routine, try something new.

WEIGHT LOSS

One of the most important things you can do for your good health is lose weight, if you need to. Sometimes, losing just 10 pounds will improve your blood glucose control. Your diabetes care provider or dietitian can help you decide how much weight loss would be good for you and help you make a weight-loss plan.

The only way to lose weight is to eat less and exercise more. And the only way to keep the weight off is to keep up these two new habits for the rest of your healthy life. A steady loss of 1 pound a week is the safest way to reach your weight-loss goal.

Ways to Eat Less

"Eat less" actually means "eat fewer calories." You may need to eat smaller portions. Or, you may be able to eat the same amount of food, if you eat foods that are lower in calories. Fat has more than twice as many calories as carbohydrate or protein. So if you eat less fat and more carbohydrate and protein, you will get fewer calories. For more on eating in this way, see HEALTHY EATING on page 36.

Food Tips

- Serve food in the kitchen. Leave the food there instead of putting it on the table. Going for seconds won't be as easy.
- Eat slowly and stop when you just begin to feel full. That way you won't get too full.
- Don't watch TV, read, or listen to the radio while you eat. These activities may draw your attention away from how much you are eating and whether you are full.
- Ask another family member to put leftovers away. That way you won't be tempted to eat the remaining food.
- Brush your teeth right after you eat. This gets the taste of food out of your mouth and may get the thought of food out of your head.
- Don't go grocery shopping when you are hungry. You may buy too much. Or you may buy things that aren't on your meal plan.
- Write out a grocery list before you go shopping. Buy just what is on the list.
- Store food out of sight.
- Eat something before you go to a social function. That way, you'll be less likely to overeat fatty foods.
- Don't skip a meal. You may overeat at your next one.
- Don't forbid yourself to eat certain foods. You'll only want them more. Try to cut down on the size of the serving or the number of times you eat that food in a week. Remember, it's the first bite that tastes best. Savor it.

Ways to Exercise More

Exercise takes weight off by helping you burn calories. If you exercise regularly, your muscles will continue to burn calories even while you're at rest. Different exercises burn different numbers of calories. Some good exercises for weight loss are cross-country skiing, walking, swimming, bicycling, and low-impact aerobics.

It's best to exercise at a moderate pace so you can keep going for a long time. If you exercise at a high pace, you will tire yourself out before you have a chance to burn enough calories. The longer you exercise, the more calories you burn. Start with a

5-minute walk each day. Add 5 minutes to the walk at the beginning of the week. Build up to where you can walk for 45 to 60 minutes. Try to do that 4 or more times a week.

To burn even more calories, add physical activities throughout the day. Walk, don't drive. Take the stairs, not the elevator. Play with the kids. Work in your garden. Go out bowling or dancing instead of watching TV.

Motivating Tips

- Don't worry about your weight. You will replace fat tissue with muscle. Muscle weighs more than fat.
- Check your measurements with a tape measure. You'll be able to see that you're getting leaner.
- For more motivating tips, see **How to Stick With It** above.

How to Keep the Weight Off

When you reach your weight-loss goal, you are faced with another challenge. Keeping weight off is even more difficult than losing it. Most people regain the weight they lost. Many people gain back even more. This happens because people go back to their old eating and exercise habits after they lose weight. To maintain your healthy weight, keep up your new habits.

Weight-Loss Clinics

If you are considering a weight-loss clinic, consult your diabetes care provider before you begin. Be sure the program has a medical doctor or nurse practitioner, a psychologist, and an exercise physiologist on staff. Look for programs that specialize in helping people with diabetes. Choose a program that

- Teaches you about nutrition and healthy food choices.
- Includes regular follow-up visits for evaluation.
- Increases your physical activity.
- Helps you learn ways to replace old habits with new, healthier ones.

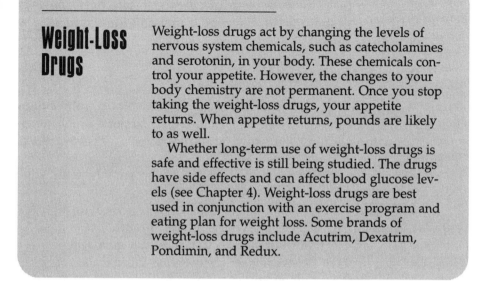

Weight-Loss Drugs

Weight-loss drugs act by changing the levels of nervous system chemicals, such as catecholamines and serotonin, in your body. These chemicals control your appetite. However, the changes to your body chemistry are not permanent. Once you stop taking the weight-loss drugs, your appetite returns. When appetite returns, pounds are likely to as well.

Whether long-term use of weight-loss drugs is safe and effective is still being studied. The drugs have side effects and can affect blood glucose levels (see Chapter 4). Weight-loss drugs are best used in conjunction with an exercise program and eating plan for weight loss. Some brands of weight-loss drugs include Acutrim, Dexatrim, Pondimin, and Redux.

DENTAL CARE

Having diabetes puts you at risk for gum disease and other mouth infections. Infections can make your blood glucose level go up. And a high blood glucose level can make mouth infections even worse. You can protect yourself by knowing the signs of gum disease and other mouth infections and by knowing how to take care of your teeth.

Gum Disease

Gum disease starts when a sticky film of bacteria, called plaque, forms on your teeth and at your gum line. You need to brush and floss your teeth to remove the plaque, or it hardens into tartar. Plaque and tartar can make your gums red, sore, and swollen and cause them to bleed when you brush or floss. This is called *gingivitis*. If you ignore gingivitis, gum disease can get worse.

Your gums may begin to pull away from your teeth. Pockets may form between your teeth and gums and fill with bacteria and pus. This is called *periodontitis*. Periodontitis can destroy your jaw bone. Your teeth may start to move. You may notice a change in the way your teeth fit when you bite or in the way your partial dentures fit. Your teeth may get loose, fall out, or have to be pulled.

Other Mouth Infections

Mouth infections affect small areas in your mouth rather than your whole mouth. They can be caused by bacteria or a fungus. Know the warning signs of mouth infections:

- Swelling around your teeth or gums or anywhere in your mouth
- Pus around your teeth or gums or anywhere in your mouth
- White or red patches anywhere in your mouth
- Pain in your mouth or sinuses that does not go away
- Dark spots or holes on your teeth
- Teeth that hurt when you eat something cold, hot, or sweet
- Pain when chewing

How to Protect Your Teeth

Control Your Blood Glucose

If you keep your blood glucose at healthy levels, you'll lower your risk of gum disease and other mouth infections.

Keep Your Teeth Clean

Brush your teeth with a fluoride toothpaste at least twice a day. Better yet, brush after every meal. Be careful not to brush too hard. You may wear away your gums. A soft toothbrush with rounded or polished bristles is easiest on your gums. Be sure to replace your toothbrush every 3 or 4 months, or sooner if the bristles are worn. One brushing technique recommended by the American Dental Association includes these steps:

1. Place the brush at a 45-degree angle to where the teeth meet the gums.
2. Gently move the brush back and forth in short strokes on the outer tooth surfaces.

3. Brush the inner tooth surfaces. Use the tip of the brush for the inner front tooth surfaces.
4. Brush the chewing surfaces.
5. Brush the upper surface of your tongue.

Floss your teeth at least once a day. If you don't like to use floss, try interdental picks or sticks. Here are flossing tips from the American Dental Association:

1. Break off about 18 inches of floss, and wind most of it around one of your middle fingers.
2. Wind the remaining floss around the same finger of the other hand. This finger will take up the floss as it is used.
3. Hold the floss tightly between your thumb and forefingers, with about 1 inch of floss between them. Use a gentle "sawing motion" to guide the floss between your teeth.
4. When the floss reaches the gum line, curve it into a C-shape against one tooth. Gently slide it into the space between the gum and the tooth until you feel resistance.
5. Hold the floss against the tooth. Gently scrape the side of the tooth, moving the floss away from the gum.

Flossing or using dental picks cleans plaque and bits of food from between your teeth. Brushing removes plaque and bits of food from the surfaces of your teeth. Ask your dentist or dental hygienist to check your brushing and flossing techniques.

See Your Dentist

Have your dentist or dental hygienist clean your teeth every 6 months. These cleanings get rid of plaque and tartar. Make sure your dentist takes complete mouth X rays every 2 years to check for bone loss. For some people, bone loss is the only sign of periodontitis.

Besides seeing your dentist for regular checkups, consult your dentist if you have any of the signs of gum disease or other mouth infections.

SKIN CARE

People with diabetes are more likely to get skin infections caused by bacteria or fungus. Diabetes can also cause some special skin problems, including diabetic dermopathy and digital sclerosis.

Bacterial Infections

Three bacterial infections that people with diabetes get more easily than people without diabetes are sties, boils, and carbuncles. All three are most often caused by staphylococcal bacteria. All appear as red, painful, pus-filled lumps.

A stye is an infected gland of the eyelid. A boil is an infected hair root or skin gland. A carbuncle is a cluster of boils. Boils and carbuncles often occur at the back of your neck, armpits, groin, or buttocks. If you think you have a stye, boil, carbuncle, or other bacterial infection, consult your diabetes care provider.

Fungal Infections

Four fungal infections that people with diabetes get more easily than people without diabetes are jock itch, athlete's foot, ringworm, and vaginal infections. Jock itch is a red, itchy area that spreads from your genitals outward over the inside of your thigh. In athlete's foot, the skin between your toes becomes itchy and sore and may crack and peel or blister.

Ringworm is a ring-shaped, red, scaly patch that may itch or blister. It can appear on the feet, groin, scalp, nails, or body. Vaginal infections are caused by the fungus *Candida albicans*. It causes a thick white discharge from the vagina and/or itching, burning, or irritation. If you think you have a fungal infection, call your diabetes care provider.

Diabetic Dermopathy

Some people with diabetes get a skin condition called diabetic dermopathy. It causes red or brown scaly patches to form, usually on the front of your legs. The spots will disappear on their own; however new spots often appear nearby. Diabetic dermopathy is harmless and needs no treatment. If you prefer to disguise its appearance, apply a heavy makeup to the legs.

Digital Sclerosis

People with diabetes may also get digital sclerosis. Digital sclerosis causes the skin on your hands, fingers, or toes to become thick and tight and look waxy or shiny. It can also cause aching and stiffness in your fingers. It may even limit movement so that you cannot easily bring the palms of your hands together, as if praying. There is no treatment for digital sclerosis, although pain killers and anti-inflammatory drugs can relieve aching joints.

How to Care for Your Skin

Keep your diabetes in good control. High blood glucose levels make it easier for you to get bacterial and fungal infections. High blood glucose levels also tend to give you dry skin.

Keep your skin clean. Take warm, not hot, baths or showers. Hot water can dry out your skin.

Keep dry parts of your skin moist. Use moisturizers and moisturizing soaps. Keep your home more humid during cold, dry months. Drink plenty of water. It helps keep your skin moist, too.

Keep other parts of your skin dry. Areas where skin touches skin need to be kept dry. These areas are between your toes, under your arms, and at your groin. Using powder on these areas can help keep them dry.

Protect your skin from the sun. The sun can dry and burn your skin. When you are out in the sun, wear a waterproof, sweatproof sunscreen with an SPF (sun protection factor) of at least 15. Wearing a hat also helps.

Treat minor skin problems. Over-the-counter products can be used to treat minor skin problems. But it's best to check with your diabetes care provider before using any skin treatment.

See a skin doctor. If you are prone to skin problems, ask your diabetes care provider about adding a skin doctor (dermatologist) to your health care team.

FOOT CARE

People with diabetes can get many kinds of foot problems. Even minor ones can quickly turn into serious ones.

Corns and Calluses

Calluses are areas of thick skin caused by regular or prolonged pressure or friction. A corn is a callus on a toe. Corns and calluses can develop on your feet when your body weight is borne unevenly. There are several things you can do to prevent calluses from forming:

Wear shoes that fit. Shoes that fit are comfortable when you buy them. Almost all new shoes are a little stiff at the start and mold to your feet with wear, but this is different from buying the wrong size and trying to break them in. Make sure there is room for you to move your toes.

Wear shoes with low heels and thick soles. Thick soles will cushion and protect your feet. Low heels distribute your weight more evenly.

Try padded socks. They not only cushion and protect feet but also reduce pressure. Be sure your shoe is large enough to fit this thicker sock. You may need extra-deep shoes.

Try shoe inserts. Ask your diabetes care provider or foot doctor about shoe inserts to better distribute your weight onto your feet.

If you get a callus or corn, have it trimmed by your diabetes care provider or foot doctor. Trying to cut corns or calluses yourself can lead to infections. Trying to remove them with over-the-counter chemicals can burn your skin. Untrimmed calluses can get very thick, break down, and turn into ulcers. And ulcers are not something you want.

Foot Ulcers

Foot ulcers are open sores or holes in the skin. Ulcers form most often over the ball of the foot or on the bottom of the big toe. Ulcers can be caused by a cut, callus, or blister that is not taken care of. Ulcers on the sides of a foot are usually caused by shoes that don't fit well. You can prevent ulcers by

- Wearing shoes that fit.
- Wearing new shoes for just a few hours at a time.
- Throwing away worn-out shoes and sneakers.
- Wearing socks that fit.
- Wearing socks without seams, holes, or bumpy areas in them.
- Putting on clean socks each day.
- Pulling or rolling your socks on gently.
- Checking for pebbles or other objects before you put on your shoes.

An ulcer can be very painful. But if you have nerve damage (see below), you may not feel it. Even though you may not feel any pain from an ulcer, you need to get medical attention right away. Walking on an ulcer can cause it to become larger and infected. An infected ulcer can lead to gangrene and amputation (see Chapter 5).

Poor Circulation

Poor circulation can make your feet feel cold and look blue or swollen. The best way to treat cold feet is to wear warm socks, even to bed. Do not use hot water bottles, heating pads, or electric blankets. They may burn your feet without you noticing. Keep your feet out of water that is too hot. Test it first with your elbow. If your feet are swollen, try lace-up shoes. You can tighten or loosen them to fit the shape of your feet.

To increase blood flow to your feet, start exercising (with your health provider's approval). Avoid sitting with your legs crossed, which can interfere with blood flow. If you smoke, stop now. Smoking limits blood flow to your feet.

Nerve Damage (Neuropathy)

Nerve damage can make your feet less able to feel pain, heat, and cold. If you have lost some of the feeling in your feet, don't go barefoot. You could hurt your foot and not notice it. If you are going swimming or wading, wear footwear made for water. Also, check your shoes before you put them on. Make sure there are no stones, nails, paper clips, pins, or other sharp objects in them. Be sure the inside of the shoe is smooth and free of tears or rough edges.

Nerve damage can affect the nerves that cause sweating. As a result, your feet may become dry and scaly, and the skin may peel and crack. If your feet have become dry and scaly, use a moisturizer twice a day. But don't put the moisturizer between your toes, because the extra moisture can lead to infection. And don't soak your feet. Soaking dries out your skin.

Nerve damage can also deform your feet. Your toes may curl up, the ball of your foot may stick out more, and your arch may get higher. These changes can cause some parts of your feet to bear more weight. Those areas are then more likely to get calluses and corns. If the shape of your feet has changed, ask your diabetes care provider or foot doctor about shoe inserts or special shoes.

How to Care for Your Feet

Check both your feet each day. Look all over them. If you cannot see well, have a friend or relative who can see well do it for you. Compare one foot to the other. Use a mirror to help see the bottom of your feet. Look for cuts, blisters, scratches, ingrown toenails, changes in color, changes in shape, punctures, anything that wasn't there the day before.

Keep your feet clean. Wash and dry them well. Don't forget to dry between your toes.

Keep your toenails trimmed. Trim your toenails to follow the curve of your toe. If you can't trim them yourself, have a member of your health care team do it.

Have your feet checked regularly. Take your shoes and socks off at every regular office visit to remind your health care provider to check your feet. Have your diabetes care provider check your feet for blood vessel, muscle, and nerve damage at least once a year.

Keep your blood glucose in control. If blood glucose levels are high, you are more likely to get foot problems.

Keep your diabetes care provider informed. Call your provider if you have a foot problem, no matter how minor.

SICK DAYS

Being sick with a cold or the flu can upset your diabetes care plan. You may not be able to eat as you usually do or take your usual diabetes pills or insulin. When you are sick, your blood glucose levels may go up too high or down too low.

Your health care team can help you make a sick-day plan before you get sick. Your sick-day plan will include what medicines to take, what to eat and drink, how often to test your blood glucose, when to call your diabetes care provider, and what to tell him or her.

What Medicines to Take

If you control your diabetes with diet and exercise or with diabetes pills, your health care provider may want you to take

What About Flu Shots and Pneumonia Shots?

People with diabetes are 4 times as likely to die from the flu or pneumonia as people without diabetes. Most people with diabetes are advised to get a flu shot once a year. The shot makes it harder to catch the flu, and even if you do catch the flu, your symptoms will likely be milder. If you are allergic to eggs, do not get a flu shot. Ask your health care provider about getting a flu shot. Also ask about getting a pneumonia shot. Many people with diabetes need one every 5 or 6 years.

regular (short-acting) insulin when you are sick. If you control your diabetes with insulin, your health care provider will most likely want you to keep taking your insulin, even if you can't keep food down. Only your diabetes care provider can tell you for sure what to do.

You may decide to take other kinds of medicines to care for your sickness. Some of these medicines may raise your blood glucose level and others may lower it. Ask your diabetes care provider or pharmacist whether the medicines you plan to take will affect your blood glucose level (see also pp. 80–81).

What to Eat and Drink

Eat foods from your usual meal plan if you can. If you can't eat your usual foods, follow your sick-day meal plan. It will include foods that are easy on your stomach. You may want to set aside a small area of your cupboard for sick-day foods. Try to eat a food with about 15 grams of carbohydrate in it every hour (see list of sick-day foods and fluids below).

If you have a fever, are vomiting, or have diarrhea, you may lose too much fluid. Try to drink a cup of fluid each hour. If your blood glucose level is over 240 mg/dl, drink sugar-free liquids

SICK-DAY FOODS AND FLUIDS WITH ~15G CARBOHYDRATE

6 saltine crackers	½ cup ice cream
5 vanilla wafers	½ cup cooked cereal
4 ounces tofu	½ cup mashed potatoes
3 graham crackers	⅓ can regular soft drink
1 fruit juice bar	⅓ cup cooked rice
1 slice toast or bread	⅓ cup fruit-flavored yogurt
1 ounce cheese	⅓ cup frozen yogurt
1 scrambled egg	¼ cup sherbet
1 cup soup	¼ cup applesauce
1 cup low-fat milk	¼ cup pudding
1 cup sports drink	¼ cup canned fruit
½ cup fruit juice	¼ cup cottage cheese
½ cup regular gelatin	

like water, caffeine-free tea, sugar-free ginger ale, or broth (chicken, beef, or vegetable). If your blood glucose level is less than 240 mg/dl, drink liquids with about 15 grams of carbohydrate in them (see list of sick-day foods and fluids on pg. 70).

How Often to Test Your Blood Glucose

Usually, you will need to test your blood glucose more often when you are sick. The sick-day plan you work out with your diabetes care team will tell you how often to test. Your plan may have you testing your blood glucose 4 or 5 times a day.

When to Call Your Provider

Call your health care provider if

• You have been sick for 2 days, and you are not getting better.
• You have been vomiting or have had diarrhea for more than 6 hours.
• Your blood glucose level is staying above 240 mg/dl.
• Your blood glucose level is staying below 60 mg/dl.
• You have any of these signs: chest pain, trouble breathing, fruity breath, or dry and cracked lips or tongue.
• You are not sure what to do to take care of yourself.

What to Tell Your Provider

Keep written records so you can tell your diabetes care provider

• How long you have been sick
• What medicines you have taken and how much
• Whether you have been able to eat and drink and how much
• Whether you are vomiting or have diarrhea
• Whether you have lost weight
• Your temperature
• Your blood glucose levels

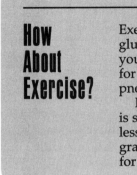

How About Exercise?

Exercising when you are sick can make your blood glucose levels go down too low or up too high. If you exercise when you are sick, it may take longer for you to get better. You may even get bronchitis or pneumonia. Do not exercise when you are sick.

Find out from your health care provider when it is safe to start exercising again. Because you may be less fit after being sick, ease into your exercise program. You might try exercising at a lower intensity, for a shorter time, or on fewer days.

Know where to reach members of your health care team or their backups on weekends, holidays, and evenings. If you must talk to someone other than a member of your health care team, be sure to tell him or her about your diabetes.

PREGNANCY

Despite your diabetes, your chances of having a healthy baby are great if you have good diabetes control before and during pregnancy and if you receive good medical care. If your diabetes control is not good before and during pregnancy, your baby may develop birth defects, become very large, or have difficulty breathing, low blood glucose, or jaundice—a yellowing of the skin. Although most of these conditions can be treated, preventing them in the first place is better for both you and your baby.

How to Ensure Your Baby's Health

Get your blood glucose in good control before pregnancy. If your blood glucose is in poor control, try to bring it into good control 3 to 6 months before you plan to get pregnant. If you wait until you know you are pregnant, your baby could already be harmed.

Keep your blood glucose in good control during your pregnancy. This will require more frequent blood glucose testing—

sometimes up to 8 times a day. It will also help you and your health care provider adjust your insulin dosage and/or meal plan.

Get fit before you get pregnant. Exercising before pregnancy may increase your endurance, help lower your blood glucose, help you lose weight, and build strength and flexibility.

Exercise during your pregnancy. Pregnancy is not the time to start a vigorous exercise program, but you will most likely be able to continue an exercise you were doing regularly before pregnancy. If you were not exercising regularly before pregnancy, ask your obstetrician about exercises that would be safe for you and your baby. Some good exercises for pregnant women include walking, low-impact aerobics, swimming, and water aerobics.

Follow your pregnancy meal plan. Your health care provider or dietitian can help you figure out what foods you need to eat to meet the demands of pregnancy. A pregnancy meal plan is designed to help you avoid high and low blood glucose while providing what your baby needs to grow. Three meals and three snacks a day are often the rule. Occasionally, a middle-of-the-night snack may be necessary. It may even be necessary to meet with your dietitian every 3 months or so during the pregnancy to keep up with your body's and the baby's needs.

Questions You May Have

Should I Still Take My Diabetes Pills?

No. Diabetes pills are not used during pregnancy because they may cause birth defects and low blood glucose in your baby. Stop taking them before you get pregnant. You can try to gain good enough control without the pills or start treatment with insulin.

If I Already Take Insulin, Will I Need More?

Most likely. You may need 2 or 3 times more insulin than usual during pregnancy, especially toward the end of pregnancy. This is normal. But do not change your insulin dosage without advice from your health care provider.

What About Alcohol, Drugs, and Other Medications?

Many medications can be harmful to your baby. Check with your health care provider before taking any prescription or over-the-counter medications.

Avoid drinking alcohol when you are pregnant and even when you are trying to conceive. And don't smoke cigarettes or use illegal drugs when pregnant. All of these may seriously harm your baby.

Is It Okay to Breastfeed?

Yes. Breastfeeding can be a wonderful experience for you and your baby. You are giving your baby antibodies (protection against infection) and an allergy-proof formula that no canned formula can duplicate.

You will probably find yourself hungrier and thirstier than normal. Therefore, you'll need a breastfeeding meal plan designed to give you and your baby the necessary nutrients.

Breastfeeding may affect your blood glucose control. So, you'll probably have to continue to test your blood glucose level more often while you are breastfeeding. You may find you have erratic blood glucose levels and more low blood glucose. On the other hand, you may find your diabetes is easier to control, and you may be able to eat a little more and take less medication. Your health care provider will help you make adjustments to your medication.

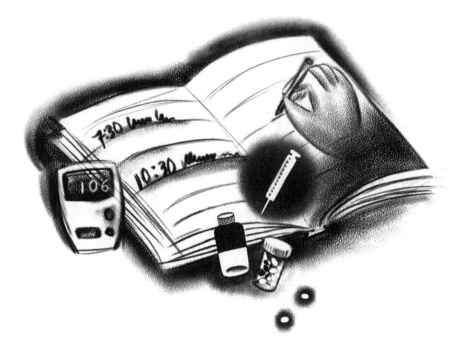

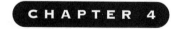

CHAPTER 4

MEDICATIONS AND MONITORING

MEDICATIONS AND MONITORING

Healthy eating and regular exercise are the first line of treatments for type 2 diabetes. If these treatments do not keep your blood glucose where you want it to be, your diabetes care provider may prescribe diabetes medications. Diabetes medications come in two forms: pills and insulin.

DIABETES PILLS

Diabetes pills generally work best for people who have had type 2 diabetes for less than 10 years. Your diabetes care provider may consider putting you on a diabetes pill when

- Your blood glucose levels before breakfast are over 126 mg/dl.
- Your blood glucose levels before bedtime are over 160 mg/dl.
- Your HbA_{1c} is above the top of the normal range.

There are five different classes of diabetes pills prescribed in the United States: sulfonylureas, biguanides, alpha-glucosidase inhibitors, thiazolidinediones, and meglitinides.

Sulfonylureas

Most diabetes pills belong to the class of drugs called sulfonylureas. There are seven different sulfonylureas available in the United States (see table on p. 78).

Sulfonylureas help your body send out more of its own insulin. They also help your body respond to insulin. And they stop your liver from putting stored glucose into your blood. These actions lower your blood glucose. Sometimes, sulfonylureas make your blood glucose go too low—for example, if you skip meals or drink too much alcohol. They may also make it easier for you to gain weight.

Possible side effects of sulfonylureas include nausea, vomiting, a skin rash, and itching. Tell your diabetes care provider about any changes you notice in your body after you start taking sulfonylureas. Do not take sulfonylureas if you are pregnant, have allergies to sulfa drugs, or have severe liver or kidney disease.

Biguanides

The biguanide metformin (brand name Glucophage) is an intermediate-acting pill that is taken 2 or 3 times a day. Metformin causes your liver to release stored glucose more slowly. It may also help your body respond to insulin. These actions keep your blood glucose levels more even. Metformin does not help your body send out more insulin. Because of this, there is less chance of low blood glucose and weight gain.

Possible side effects of metformin include a metallic taste in your mouth, an upset stomach, nausea, loss of appetite, and diarrhea. These side effects usually go away after a short time. If you have heart, kidney, or liver disease, do not take metformin, because it can cause you to develop lactic acidosis—a life-threatening buildup of acid in the blood.

Alpha-Glucosidase Inhibitors

The alpha-glucosidase inhibitors acarbose (brand name Precose) and miglitol (brand name Glyset) are short-acting pills taken 3 times a day, with main meals. These drugs work by slowing

SULFONYLUREAS			
Generic Name	**Brand Name**	**Action Time**	**Doses Per Day**
Acetohexamide	Dymelor	Intermediate	1 or 2
Chlorpropamide	Diabinese	Long	1
Glipizide	Glucotrol	Intermediate	1 or 2
	Glucotrol XL	Long	
Glimepiride	Amaryl	Long	1
Glyburide	Diaßeta	Intermediate	1 or 2
	Micronase		
	Glynase		
	PresTab		
Tolazamide	Tolinase	Intermediate	1 or 2
Tolbutamide	Orinase	Short	2 or 3

the time it takes for your intestine to break down food into glucose. This causes glucose to enter your blood more slowly. Your blood glucose then stays more even, with fewer highs and lows. Acarbose and miglitol are especially helpful at flattening out the sharp rise in glucose that may occur after meals.

Possible side effects of alpha-glucosidase inhibitors include gas, bloating, and diarrhea. Most people get these side effects when they first begin using the drugs, then after a while, the side effects go away. But some people will still have them. Do not take acarbose or miglitol if you have any gastrointestinal diseases.

Thiazolidinediones

The thiazolidinediones rosiglitazone (brand name Avandia) and pioglitazone (brand name Actos) are approved for use in people with type 2 diabetes who are taking insulin. (A third thiazolidinedione, troglitazone—brand name Rezulin—was withdrawn from the market in March 2000 because it was found to cause liver problems.) People with type 2 diabetes who take these drugs may be able to reduce their insulin doses. Thiazolidinediones enhance the action of insulin so that your body needs less. They have also been shown to lower triglyceride levels and raise HDL (the good) cholesterol levels. Because they may cause fluid retention, these drugs are not recommended for people with heart disease.

Meglitinides

The meglitinide repaglinide (brand name Prandin) is usually prescribed for people whose type 2 diabetes can't be controlled by diet and exercise alone. (The meglitinide natiglinide— brand name Starlix—is in development; it should be on the market by early 2001.) Repaglinide differs from other diabetes pills in that it works very quickly and is taken just prior to eating—anytime from 30 minutes before meals to right before you eat. Repaglinide works by increasing the amount of insulin your body releases during and just after a meal. This results in smaller meal-related increases in blood glucose. Because repaglinide is eliminated from the bloodstream within three to four hours, it does not cause your body to continuously release insulin for long periods of time.

Possible side effects of repaglinide include low blood glucose, upper respiratory infections, nausea, diarrhea, constipation, joint pain, and headache. Do not take repaglinide if you are pregnant, have type 1 diabetes, or have type 2 and your body is no longer producing insulin.

Diabetes pills do not take the place of diet and exercise. They work with them. In fact, if you do not follow your meal and exercise plans, diabetes pills may not work for you.

Sometimes, diabetes pills work for a little while, then stop working. This often happens after several years. If your diabetes pills stop working, your diabetes care provider may put you on another pill, two different types of pills, a pill and insulin, or insulin alone.

You and your diabetes care provider will need to work together to find the best treatment. It will be important for you to keep records of when you take your medication and the dosage. You may need to test your blood glucose more often until your diabetes care provider finds the right doses for you.

MEDICATIONS THAT CAN AFFECT BLOOD GLUCOSE LEVELS

Generic Name	Brand Name	Effect on Blood Glucose Level	Interacts with Diabetes Pills?	Common Uses
Alcohol	Ingredient in many medications	Lowers	Yes	Carry active ingredient in drug into metabolism
Aspirin	Many brand names	May lower if taken in large doses	Yes	Treat general pain or fever; treat arthritis
Beta-blockers	Inderal Sectral Tenormin Lopressor Visken Blocadren	May mask low blood glucose	Yes	Treat high blood pressure, angina, unsteady heartbeat, overactive thyroid, and other ailments
Chloramphenicol	Chloromycetin	Lowers*	Yes	Treat bacterial infections
Clofibrate	Atromid-S	Lowers*	Yes	Treat high cholesterol and triglyceride levels
Diazoxide	Hyperstat Proglycem	Raises	Yes	Treat low blood glucose caused by tumors in pancreas; sometimes used to treat high blood pressure
Diuretics	Diuril HydroDIURIL Edecrin Esidrix Diamox Lasix Hygroton	May raise if taken in high doses	Yes	Relieve fluid buildup by increasing amount of water in urine
Epinephrine	Epinephrine	Raises	Yes	Revive heartbeat; treat severe allergic reactions
Epinephrine-like drugs (ephedrine, pseudoephedrine phenylephrine)	Many cold, flu, and allergy medicines	Raises	Yes	Treat runny noses, flu, allergies, colds
Estrogens, birth control pills	Many brand names	May raise	No	Prevent pregnancy; lessen the effects of menopause

continued

MEDICATIONS THAT CAN AFFECT BLOOD GLUCOSE LEVELS (CONT)

Generic Name	Brand Name	Effect on Blood Glucose Level	Interacts with Diabetes Pills?	Common Uses
Lithium carbonate	Eskalith Lithonate	Raises	No	Treat manic depression
Methyldopa	Aldomet	Lowers*	Yes	Treat high blood pressure
Monoamine oxidase (MAO) inhibitors	Parnate Nardil	Lowers	Yes	Treat severe depression
Nicotinic acid, niacin	Nicolar Nicobid	Raises	No	Treat nutrient deficiency; treat high cholesterol levels
Phenobarbital	Many brand names	Raises*	Yes	Sedate; treat epilepsy
Phentermine	Several brand names	Raises	Yes	Suppress appetite
Phenylbutazone	Butazolidin	Lowers*	Yes	Treat arthritis
Phenylpropanol-amine	Acutrim Dexatrim	Raises	Yes	Suppress appetite
Phenytoin	Dilantin	Raises	Yes	Treat epilepsy and other nervous system disorders
Rifampin	Rifadin	Raises*	Yes	Treat tuberculosis
Steroids (prednisone, cortisone, dexamethasone)	Steraspred Deltasone Cortone Decadron	Raises	Yes	Reduce inflammation, redness, and swelling
Sulfa drugs	Gantrisin Septra Bactrim	Lowers*	Yes	Treat bacterial infections
Thyroid preparations	Armour S-P-T	Raises	No	Treat lessened or absent thyroid function

*These drugs raise or lower blood glucose only when used in combination with diabetes pills.

OTHER MEDICATIONS

You may take other prescription or over-the-counter medications. It's important to know how these medications act inside your body and how they interact with each other. Some medications may lower or raise your blood glucose level or interfere with how your body uses diabetes pills (see pp. 80–81).

Be sure to follow all instructions for taking your medications. Make sure all members of your health care team know what medications you are taking. Try to use a single pharmacy for all your prescriptions. That way, all your medications can be listed on one record. Test your blood glucose to see whether a new medication affects your blood glucose level. If you find that a medication you are taking greatly upsets your blood glucose control, ask your diabetes care provider or pharmacist about it.

INSULIN

In type 2 diabetes, your body doesn't make enough insulin, or your body has a hard time using the insulin, or both. You may need to take extra insulin.

There are two different sources of insulin: animals and bacteria. Animal (pork or pork/beef) insulin comes from the pancreases of dead pigs and cows. Human insulin is made by putting the human gene for insulin into bacteria, causing the bacteria to make human insulin. The insulin is then extracted and purified.

Insulin Types

There are several types of insulin. They are grouped by the way they act in the body. Insulin's action has three parts: onset, peak time, and duration. Onset is how long insulin takes to start working. Peak time is when insulin is working its hardest. Duration is how long insulin keeps working.

INSULIN ACTION				
	Rapid-Acting Insulin	Short-Acting Insulin	Intermediate-Acting Insulin	Long-Acting Insulin
Onset	20-40 minutes	30-60 minutes	2-4 hours	6-14 hours
Peak	30-120 minutes	1-3 hours	4-14 hours	14-24 hours
Duration	4-6 hours	5-7 hours	18-24 hours	20-36 hours
Types	Lispro	Regular	NPH and Lente	Ultralente

The times for onset, peak, and duration are given as ranges in the table on p. 82. There are two reasons for these ranges: 1) insulin may work slower or faster in you than in someone else, and 2) human insulin works faster than animal insulin.

Insulin Strengths

Insulins come in different strengths. The most common strength of insulin used in the United States is U-100 insulin. This means that there are 100 units of insulin per milliliter of fluid. U-500 insulin is also available in the United States. If you inject insulin, the syringe must match the strength of your insulin. For instance, if you use U-100 insulin, use a U-100 syringe.

Insulin Mixtures

Different combinations of insulins can be mixed by you or bought premixed. Regular insulins mix easily with NPH insulins. Such mixtures can be made several days in advance and stored in syringes in the refrigerator. Or you can inject these mixed insulins right away. The potency of regular insulin does not last long when mixed with lente or ultralente insulins. Therefore, it is best to inject mixtures of regular and lente or ultralente immediately after mixing.

Insulin Storage and Safety

Insulin makers advise storing your insulin in the refrigerator. Do not put your insulin in the freezer or allow it to warm in the sun or in a hot car. Extreme temperatures can destroy insulin. The vial of insulin you are using can be left at room temperature for up to a month. Carry it so that it won't get bumped and jostled a lot. Otherwise, it will lose potency.

Check the expiration date before opening your insulin. If the date has passed, don't use the insulin. If the date is yet to come, look closely at the insulin in the vial. Regular insulin should be clear, with no floating pieces or color. NPH, lente, and ultralente insulin should be cloudy but without floating pieces or crystals. If the insulin does not look as it should, return the unopened vial of insulin to the place you bought it for an exchange or refund.

Insulin Injections

Insulin needs to be put under the skin, in the fat, to work well. One way to get insulin under the skin is by using syringes with needles. You may have to try several brands of syringes before you find one that suits you. Pick a syringe that is

- Made to hold the strength (such as U-100) of insulin you use.
- Large enough to hold your entire dose for each injection; for example, if you take 45 units, you cannot use a 30-unit syringe.
- Easy to read. The markings on the syringe may be easier to read if the plunger is a different color.
- Comfortable. Today's syringes have tiny needles with a slick coating so that they go in easily. Try several brands to find the ones most comfortable to you.

Filling a Syringe with Insulin

To fill a syringe with insulin, you will need a sterile disposable syringe with needle, a vial of insulin, a bottle of 70% isopropyl alcohol, a cotton ball or cotton swab or gauze, and something clean to set the filled syringe on if you need to put it down.

1. Wash your hands with soap and water.
2. Gently roll the vial of insulin in your hands to mix the insulin. (You do not need to do this to rapid- or short-acting insulin.)
3. Wipe the top of the insulin vial with alcohol. Let the alcohol dry completely (don't blow on it to dry it).
4. Draw air into the syringe. Stop at the mark for the insulin dose you want. Put the needle in the vial and inject the air into it.
5. Turn the vial upside down and draw insulin into the syringe. Stop at the mark for the number of units you want.
6. Remove the needle from the vial.
7. Check for air bubbles on the inside of the syringe. If there are air bubbles, flick your forefinger against the upright syringe a couple of times to get them out.
8. If you need to set the syringe down, place it on its side, and make sure the needle doesn't touch anything.

Filling a Syringe with Two Kinds of Insulin

To fill a syringe with two kinds of insulin (called an insulin mixture), you will need a sterile disposable syringe with needle, two vials of insulin, a bottle of 70% isopropyl alcohol, a cotton ball or cotton swab or gauze, and something clean to set the filled syringe on if you need to put it down.

1. Wash your hands with soap and water.
2. Gently roll each vial of insulin in your hands to mix the insulin. (You do not need to do this to rapid- or short-acting insulin.)
3. Wipe the top of each insulin vial with alcohol. Let the alcohol dry completely (don't blow on it to dry it).
4. Draw air into the syringe. Stop at the mark for the dose you want of your intermediate- or long-acting insulin (for instance, 30 units). Inject the air into that vial.
5. Draw air into the syringe a second time. Stop at the mark for the dose you want of your rapid- or short-acting insulin (for instance, 10 units). Inject the air into that vial.
6. With the needle still in the rapid- or short-acting insulin vial, turn the vial upside down.
7. Draw insulin into the syringe. Stop at the mark for the number of units of short-acting insulin you want.
8. Take the needle out of the rapid- or short-acting insulin vial.
9. Put the needle in the intermediate- or long-acting insulin vial, and turn the vial upside down.
10. Draw insulin into the syringe. Stop at the mark for the total number of units of insulin you want, that is, the number of units of rapid- or short-acting insulin added to the number of units of intermediate- or long-acting insulin. (To add 30 units of intermediate- or long-acting insulin to the 10 units of short-acting insulin already in the syringe, pull the plunger back to the 40-unit mark.)
11. If you pull out too much of the second insulin, throw away the insulin in your syringe and start over from the beginning.
12. Once you have the amount you want, remove the needle from the vial.
13. Check for air bubbles on the inside of the syringe. If there are air bubbles, flick your forefinger against the upright syringe a couple of times to get them out.

14. If you need to set the syringe down, place it on its side, and make sure the needle doesn't touch anything.

Where to Inject Insulin

When choosing a place to inject insulin, consider the area and the site. Areas are the places on your body where it is good to inject insulin. Four good areas are your

1. Abdomen (anywhere except within 2 inches of your navel)
2. Upper arms (outside part)
3. Buttocks (anywhere)
4. Thighs (front and outside parts, not inner thigh, not right above your knee)

These areas absorb insulin at different speeds. Your abdomen absorbs insulin the fastest, followed by the arms, thighs, and buttocks. You may prefer to inject insulin in the same area so that you know how it will act. Or you may want to choose your area according to how fast or slow you want the insulin to start working. Either way, keep track of how your body responds by testing your blood glucose and recording the results.

Now pretend that each area is covered with circles that are 1 inch apart. Each circle is one site. The number of sites you have depends on how big your body is. The bigger your body, the more sites you have in each area.

Within each area, change sites with each injection. This is called site rotation. To rotate sites, you use a different circle for each injection until all the circles have been used up. Then you start all over again. If you inject all your insulin in the same site, you can damage the tissue under your skin.

How to Inject Insulin

To inject insulin, you will need a filled sterile syringe, a bottle of 70% isopropyl alcohol, and cotton balls or gauze.

1. Wash your hands with soap and water.
2. Clean the site with alcohol.
3. Gently pinch a fold of skin between your thumb and forefinger.

4. Push the needle through the skin at a 90-degree angle. If you are thin, you may need to push the needle in at a 45-degree angle to avoid muscle.
5. After the needle is in, push in the plunger to inject the insulin.
6. Pull the needle out.
7. Cover the injection site with a dry cotton ball or gauze or your finger and apply slight pressure to the site for 5 to 8 seconds without rubbing. Rubbing may disperse the insulin too quickly or cause irritation.

How to Make the Injection More Comfortable

- Inject insulin at room temperature. Using cold insulin right from the refrigerator may make it hurt more.
- Make sure there are no air bubbles in the syringe before you inject the insulin.
- Wait until the alcohol you put on your skin is dry.
- Relax your muscles in the area.
- Puncture the skin quickly.
- Keep the needle going in the same direction when you put it in and take it out.
- Use sharp, not dull, needles.

How to Reuse Syringes

Makers of disposable syringes recommend that they be used only once. The makers cannot guarantee that the syringe will stay sterile. If you want to use your syringes more than once, check with your diabetes care provider first.

- Recap the needle after each use to keep it clean.
- Keep the needle from touching anything but clean skin and your insulin vial stopper.
- Store the used syringe at room temperature.
- Throw away the syringe when the needle is dull, has been bent, or has come into contact with any surface other than your skin.
- Don't try to clean the needle with alcohol. Alcohol may remove the slick coating that makes shots less painful.
- Watch out for infection at the site.

How to Dispose of Syringes

The best way to dispose of syringes and needles is to place them in a puncture-proof container of heavy-duty plastic or metal with a screw cap or other lid that can be sealed shut before it is placed in the garbage. Removing the needles from the syringes will prevent anyone from reusing them.

Some states require you to destroy used insulin syringes and needles. But be careful if you recap, bend, or break a needle—you or someone else could get pricked with it.

There may be special rules for getting rid of syringes and needles where you live. Ask your local garbage company or city or county waste authority what method meets their rules.

When traveling, bring your used syringes home. You can pack them in a heavy-duty container, such as a hard plastic pencil box, for transport.

By not properly disposing of your syringes, you could cause garbage collectors and other cleaning people injury and worry about exposure to HIV, AIDS, and hepatitis.

Syringe Alternatives

If you don't like the traditional needle and syringe plunger, you might want to try an infuser, an insulin pen, or a jet injector. An infuser is a needle that remains taped in place at the site for 2 or 3 days. Insulin is injected into this needle rather than through the skin. An insulin pen is like a cartridge ink pen. Instead of ink, the cartridge is filled with insulin. And instead of a writing point, there is a needle. A jet injector uses pressure instead of a needle to move insulin under your skin.

Injection Aids

If you have poor eyesight, you may want to try a syringe magnifier, which enlarges the markings on the syringe barrel, or a dose gauge, which helps you measure an accurate insulin dose (even mixed doses).

If your hands are not very steady, you might try a needle guide and/or vial stabilizer to help you insert your needle into the insulin vial to draw up your dose.

If you have lost some dexterity, you may want to consider a spring-loaded metal syringe.

Insulin Pumps

An insulin pump is a battery-powered, computerized device about the size of a deck of cards. You wear it on your belt or in your pocket. Inside the pump is a syringe of short-acting insulin with a gear-driven plunger. A thin tube, 21 to 43 inches long, is attached to the pump. At the other end of the tube is a needle or catheter. You insert the needle or catheter under your skin, usually in your abdomen or thigh, and tape it in place.

Insulin is delivered through the tube and needle or catheter into your body. You "program" the pump. You tell it how much insulin you want and when you want it.

You wear an insulin pump pretty much all the time, either inside or outside your clothes. A pump may be waterproof or come with a waterproof case for showers and swimming. You can, of course, take the pump off, for example, when you're exercising, and put it back on when you're finished.

SELF-MONITORING OF BLOOD GLUCOSE

One of the best ways to keep track of how well your diabetes care plan is working is to test your blood glucose. Instead of simply saying to yourself, "I feel fine" or "I feel lousy," you take measurements and keep records. Testing helps you find out what happens to your blood glucose level when you eat certain foods, do certain exercises, or lose weight. Testing helps you find out what happens to your blood glucose level when you take diabetes pills or insulin, are sick, or are stressed.

A blood test can help you decide what to do to take care of your diabetes. Tests may prompt you to eat a snack, take more insulin, or exercise more. Tests may alert you to treat high or low blood glucose. Records of your tests can help your health care team figure out which diabetes pills or insulin works best for you, at what dosage, and at what times.

How to Test Blood Glucose

You can test your blood glucose with either a glucose meter or test strips that you read by eye. It's important to follow the instructions that come with the product you buy. You'll need a lancet, a clean test strip, a cotton ball or tissue (with some methods), a watch or other timing device (with some methods), and a color chart or a blood glucose meter.

1. Wash your hands with soap and water.
2. Prick the side of your finger with a lancet.
3. Squeeze out a drop of blood.
4. Let the drop of blood fall on a test strip pad, if possible.
5. Wait.
6. Wipe off or blot excess blood, if instructed to do so, with a cotton ball or tissue.
7. Read your blood glucose number in the window on the meter or match the color of the strip to a color chart to find your glucose range.
8. Dispose of the lancet the same way as your syringe needles.
9. Record your finding.

When to Test Blood Glucose

Your diabetes care provider can help you figure out when to test. Testing at specific times can be useful. For instance, a test done 1 or 2 hours after a meal lets you see how high your blood glucose rises after you eat certain kinds and amounts of foods. A test at 2 or 3 A.M. tells you if you have low blood glucose at night. There are eight test times for you to choose from:

1. Before breakfast
2. 1 to 2 hours after breakfast
3. Before lunch
4. 1 to 2 hours after lunch
5. Before supper
6. 1 to 2 hours after supper
7. Before bedtime
8. At 2 or 3 A.M.

The more you test, the more you will know about your blood glucose levels. And the more you know about your blood glucose levels, the better able you will be to get those levels where you and your health care team want them to be. Here are some test times to talk about with your health care team:

- If you treat with diet and exercise only, test before you eat breakfast and 1 or 2 hours after a meal.
- If you are taking diabetes pills, test 1 or 2 times a day. If you test once a day, do it before you eat breakfast. If you test twice a day, test first when you get up in the morning and vary the time of the second test.
- If you are taking insulin, test 2 to 4 times a day and vary the times you test.

When to Do Extra Blood Glucose Tests

Your health care team may want you to do extra blood glucose tests

- When your team is trying to find the best dose of diabetes pills or insulin for you.
- When you change your exercise program or meal plan.
- When you start a new drug that can affect your glucose level.
- When you think your glucose is low or high.
- When you are sick.
- When you are pregnant.
- When you are traveling.
- When you have been exercising for more than an hour .
- Before and after you exercise.
- Before you drive.
- Before activities that take a lot of concentration.

Keep Records

Be sure to write down your test results, date, and time. Do this even if you have a meter with a memory. Your health care team can tell you what else to record. You may be asked to record

- The foods you eat and when you eat them.
- Times that you miss meals or snacks.

- Times that you eat large or small meals.
- Times that you drink alcohol and how much you drink.
- How much you weigh.
- How much insulin or how many diabetes pills you take and when.
- When and how long you exercise.
- When and how you treat low or high blood glucose.
- When you are ill, injured, stressed, or have just had surgery.

You might find it easiest to keep all your records in one book. Your diabetes care provider can probably give you a record book. Share your records with your health care team. Together, you can make needed changes in your diabetes care plan. A better plan makes it easier for you to take care of your diabetes.

Is Your Meter Accurate?

Sometimes you may wonder whether your meter is accurate, especially if your meter gives you a reading you were not expecting or if your meter's reading and that of a lab do not match. Misreadings can occur for many reasons. The problem may be with the meter itself, the testing strips, or your testing technique.

Check the Meter

Be sure that your meter is at room temperature. Using a meter in very hot or very cold temperatures can cause inaccurate readings.

Keep your meter clean, if your meter requires it. The user's manual that came with the meter will say whether you need to clean it and how to clean it. Review the directions for cleaning your meter or call the meter's maker if you are unsure about the right way to clean your meter. Dirty meters can give false results.

Calibrate your meter each time you start a new batch of test strips. The chemical mix that is put on test strips differs a little from batch to batch. Each batch of strips may give slightly different results. Calibrating your meter means resetting it so that you still get correct answers. A few meters calibrate themselves. If you don't recall the calibration procedure and/or can't find the instructions that came with your meter, call the meter's maker. You'll find the maker's phone number on the back of most machines.

Your meter should have come with a control solution. The control solution contains a known amount of glucose. Run a test using the control solution anytime the meter does not seem to be working right. It's also a good idea to run a test when you buy the meter, when you open a new batch of test strips, and when you change the batteries. Compare the answer you get with what the meter's manual says you should get. If the answers are not close, something is wrong. The meter may be broken, or it may need a new battery. Or the problem may be with the test strips or your testing technique.

Check the Test Strips

Confirm that the test strips you have will work with your meter. Keep your test strips in a place that is cool and dry. Test strips may give false readings if they have been stored in extreme hot or cold temperatures and/or extreme humidity. Your bathroom, for example, can be too humid for test strips. And the glove compartment of your car can be too hot.

Keep test strips in the dark (in their foil or vial) until you are ready to use them. When you remove strips, close the rest up right away to avoid exposing them to direct light for any length of time.

Note the expiration date on each vial or package of test strips. Be sure to throw away test strips that are past their expiration date. Also throw them out if they don't look like fresh new strips.

Check Your Technique

Study your manual (and instruction video, if you have one) to make sure you are using your meter correctly. Take your meter to your appointments with your diabetes care provider. Have a member of your health care team check how you do the test.

Test your blood within 5 to 10 minutes of having your blood drawn at the lab. Your reading should be within 15 percent of the lab's reading. That is, if the lab reading is 200 mg/dl, your meter reading should be between 170 and 230 mg/dl: $200 \times .15$ (15 percent) = 30; $200 - 30 = 170$ and $200 + 30 = 230$.

The size of the drop of blood you use may affect the result. Some meters need larger drops of blood than others. With some meters, you must wipe the blood in a certain way and with a certain material, such as a tissue or cotton ball. Usually, you should let the blood fall onto the strip without actually touching your finger to the pad.

LOW BLOOD GLUCOSE

Low blood glucose is known as hypoglycemia. You may get low blood glucose if you use insulin or take sulfonylureas. If not treated, low blood glucose can make you pass out. At worst, low blood glucose may cause seizures, coma, and even death. There are many causes of low blood glucose.

Perhaps you ate too little food or too few carbohydrates. Maybe you delayed or skipped a meal or snack. You might have exercised harder or longer than usual. Or you may have taken too much insulin or too many diabetes pills. Perhaps you are sick or you drank alcohol on an empty stomach.

Many people experience warning signs of low blood glucose. Your own signs may be different from those someone else feels.

WARNING SIGNS

Low Blood Glucose

▪ Anger	▪ Nausea
▪ Anxiety	▪ Nervousness
▪ Blurred vision	▪ Numbness
▪ Clamminess	▪ Pallor
▪ Clumsiness	▪ Pounding heart
▪ Confusion	▪ Sadness
▪ Fatigue	▪ Shakiness
▪ Headache	▪ Sleepiness
▪ Hunger	▪ Stubbornness
▪ Impatience	▪ Sweating
▪ Irritability	▪ Tension
▪ Light-headedness	▪ Weakness

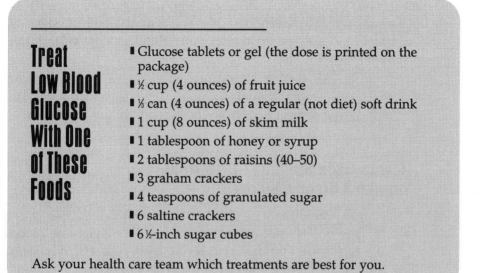

Treat Low Blood Glucose With One of These Foods

- Glucose tablets or gel (the dose is printed on the package)
- ½ cup (4 ounces) of fruit juice
- ⅓ can (4 ounces) of a regular (not diet) soft drink
- 1 cup (8 ounces) of skim milk
- 1 tablespoon of honey or syrup
- 2 tablespoons of raisins (40–50)
- 3 graham crackers
- 4 teaspoons of granulated sugar
- 6 saltine crackers
- 6 ½-inch sugar cubes

Ask your health care team which treatments are best for you.

Learn your early warning signs of low blood glucose. Tell your signs to someone who can help you watch out for them. When any of your warning signs occur, you need to treat low blood glucose right away.

How to Treat Yourself for Low Blood Glucose

1. Test your blood glucose with a meter if you can. If it is under 70 mg/dl, go to steps 2 and 3. If you can't test, go to steps 2 and 4.
2. Eat or drink something with about 15 grams (½ ounce) of carbohydrate. Foods with 15 grams of carbohydrate are listed in the table on p. 95.
3. Wait 15 to 20 minutes, then test again.

   If your blood glucose is still below 70 mg/dl, repeat steps 2 and 3. If you have repeated steps 2 and 3 and your blood glucose is still below 70 mg/dl, call your diabetes care provider, or have someone take you to a hospital emergency room. You may need help to treat your low blood glucose. Or something else may be causing the signs.

If your blood glucose is over 70 mg/dl, stop drinking and/or eating foods listed in the table. You may still feel the signs of low blood glucose even after your blood glucose is back up. Go to step 4.

4. If your next meal is more than an hour away, eat a small snack of carbohydrate and protein. Try a slice of bread with reduced-fat peanut butter or 6 crackers with low-fat cheese.

How to Have Someone Else Treat Your Low Blood Glucose

Sometimes you will not be able to treat low blood glucose yourself. Maybe you do not notice your signs. Or maybe low blood glucose has made you too confused to treat yourself. Whatever the reason, teach someone else *ahead of time* to do it.

Keep foods to treat low blood glucose near you at all times. Place a small box of juice in your desk drawer at work or at school. Put glucose tablets or gel in your purse or coat pocket and in the glove compartment of your car. Tell others where you keep them.

If you take insulin, get a glucagon emergency kit. Your diabetes care provider can prescribe one. Glucagon is a hormone that is made in the pancreas. Glucagon makes the liver release glucose into the blood.

A glucagon kit comes with a syringe of glucagon and instructions on how to use it. Keep the kit with you. Tell family, friends, and coworkers where you keep it. You or a member of your health care team can teach them how to use it.

If you can swallow
1. Have someone get you to eat or drink something with carbohydrate in it.

If you cannot swallow or if you pass out
1. Have someone inject you with glucagon in the front of the thigh or the shoulder muscle.
2. Have someone turn you on your side. This will keep you from choking if you throw up from the glucagon. (Some people feel sick to their stomach after glucagon.)

3. Once you are alert, eat a snack of carbohydrate that's easy on your stomach. Try 6 saltine crackers. Follow it up with a snack of protein, such as a slice of turkey breast or low-fat cheese.
4. Test your blood glucose every 30 to 60 minutes to make sure low blood glucose is not coming back.

If you cannot swallow and glucagon is not available OR
If you cannot swallow and nobody knows how to use glucagon
1. Have someone call 911 for an ambulance.
2. Have someone moisten his or her fingertip, dip the fingertip in table sugar, and rub his or her sugar-coated fingertip against the inside of your cheek until the sugar dissolves, being careful to keep the finger away from your teeth. (If you go into a seizure, you may bite the finger.)

OR

Have someone open a tube of cake frosting and insert the open end inside your cheek. Have the person squeeze a small amount of frosting into your mouth and massage the outside of your cheek.
3. Keep doing step 2 until the ambulance arrives.

HIGH BLOOD GLUCOSE

High blood glucose is known as hyperglycemia. High blood glucose is one of the signs of diabetes. Having high blood glucose for a long time can damage your eyes, kidneys, heart, nerves, and blood vessels.

There are many causes of high blood glucose. Maybe you ate too much food. Perhaps you took too few diabetes pills or too little insulin or did not take them at all. You might be sick or feeling stressed. Maybe you skipped your usual exercise.

WARNING SIGNS

High Blood Glucose

- Headache
- Blurry vision
- Thirst
- Hunger
- Upset stomach
- Frequent urination
- Dry, itchy skin
- Fruity smell on breath

High blood glucose is harder to sense than low blood glucose. If your glucose is very high, you may feel some of the signs listed in the table on p. 97.

You may not be able to tell that your glucose is too high by signs alone. The only sure way to know is to test your blood glucose. Your glucose reading will help you decide what to do.

If your blood glucose level is between 180 and 240 mg/dl, your provider may advise you to take a walk, do some other exercise, or have a smaller upcoming snack.

If your blood glucose level is 350 to 400 mg/dl (or another high number set by your team), call your diabetes care provider.

If your blood glucose level goes above 500 mg/dl, call your diabetes care provider and have someone take you to the hospital right away.

HHNS

HHNS is an abbreviation for hyperosmolar hyperglycemic non-ketotic syndrome. It is a life-threatening condition of high blood glucose and severe dehydration. Anyone with type 2 diabetes can develop HHNS. But HHNS doesn't just happen. It is usually brought on by something else, such as an illness, a heart attack, or extensive burns.

WARNING SIGNS

HHNS (HYPEROSMOLAR HYPERGLYCEMIC NONKETOTIC SYNDROME)

- Blood glucose level over 600 mg/dl
- Dry, parched mouth
- Extreme thirst (although this may gradually disappear)
- Warm, dry skin that does not sweat
- High fever (105°F, for example)
- Sleepiness or confusion
- Loss of vision
- Hallucinations
- Weakness on one side of your body

In HHNS, blood glucose levels rise, and your body tries to get rid of the excess glucose by passing it into your urine. This makes your urine thicker. Fluids are pulled from all over your body to thin out the urine. You make lots of urine, and you have to urinate more often. You also get very thirsty. If you don't drink enough fluids at this point, you can get dehydrated.

If HHNS continues, the severe dehydration will lead to seizures, coma, and eventually death. HHNS usually takes days or even several weeks to develop. When you are sick, drink a glassful of fluid (alcohol-free and caffeine-free) every hour, and test your blood glucose more often.

MONITORING DONE BY YOUR HEALTH CARE TEAM

Your health care team will monitor your health and how well you are doing with your diabetes care. How often you need to see members of your health care team will depend on your health, your blood glucose goals, and any changes that need to be made to your diabetes care plan. The chart on p. 100 will give you an idea of when to visit your health care providers and what tests to expect.

Most people with type 2 diabetes have two regular checkups a year. Regular checkups help your health care team detect

SAMPLE GLYCOHEMOGLOBIN MEASUREMENTS	
Glycohemoglobin by HbA$_{1c}$ Measurement	Average Blood Glucose Level (mg/dl)
4	60
5	90
6	120
7	150
8	180
9	210
10	240
11	270
12	300
13	330

RECOMMENDED FREQUENCY OF MEDICAL EXAMS AND TESTS

	Every 3 Months	Every 6 Months	Every Year	Every 2–3 Years	As Needed
Regular Visits*					
If not meeting goals	●				
If meeting goals		●			
Physical Exam			●		
Dilated Eye Exam			●		
Lipid Profile					
If last reading was abnormal			●		
If last reading was normal				●	
Glycohemoglobin Test					
If not meeting goals or if treatment changes	●				
If meeting goals		●			
Kidney Tests			●		
Urine Tests			●		
Thyroid Tests					●
Electrocardiogram					●

*Regular visits include measurement of your height, weight, and blood pressure, a foot exam, an eye exam, and a check on anything that was abnormal at a previous visit.

problems as early as possible. During a physical exam, members of your health care team will check your

- Height and weight
- Blood pressure and pulse
- Eyes
- Mouth, teeth, and gums
- Neck
- Heart
- Abdomen
- Hands and fingers
- Feet
- Skin
- Nervous system

Sometimes, your health care team will order laboratory tests, such as a glycohemoglobin test to measure your average blood glucose level for the past 2 to 4 months or a blood fat (lipid) profile to measure your total cholesterol, LDL cholesterol, HDL cholesterol, and triglycerides. (For sample glycohemoglobin measurements, see the table below; for sample lipid profile values, see the **Blood Fats (Lipid) Profile** table on p. 116 in Chapter 5.)

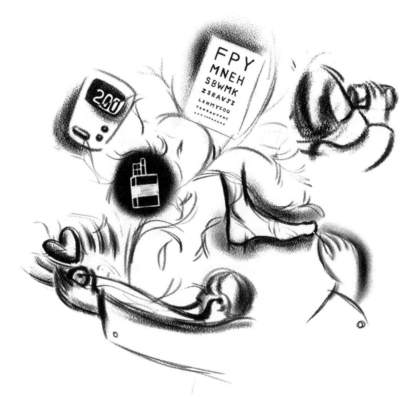

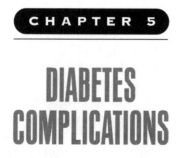

CHAPTER 5

DIABETES COMPLICATIONS

DIABETES COMPLICATIONS

Diabetes can lead to other conditions called diabetes complications. Some can develop quickly, while others appear after many years of diabetes. Complications can affect your blood vessels, heart, brain, legs and feet, eyes, kidneys, and nerves.

BLOOD VESSELS

The enemies of your blood vessels are high blood glucose, high blood pressure, and high blood fats (cholesterol and triglycerides). All can damage your blood vessels. Often, you will not notice any signs until the damage has been done.

When blood vessels are damaged, they become weak, narrow, or blocked. This is called atherosclerosis, or hardening of the arteries. Less blood flows through the blood vessels to nourish the parts of your body with oxygen. When your body parts get less oxygen, they don't work as well and can become damaged or die.

HEART

Decreased blood flow to your heart can cause pain in your chest during exertion (angina). The pain goes away after resting a minute or so. Angina is a signal that your heart muscle is working hard but getting too little blood for its effort.

Angina may be relieved by drugs (such as nitrates—including nitroglycerine—beta-blockers, calcium-channel blockers, and vasodilators) that increase the amount of oxygen going to the heart or reduce the amount of oxygen the heart needs when it's working hard. Surgery may be needed when these treatments are not working or when a heart attack is likely to occur.

Despite decreased blood flow to the heart, some people with diabetes may not have chest pain. Some may even have a severe heart attack and not feel pain. This happens when nerves to the heart have become damaged as a complication of diabetes and can't transmit pain.

A heart attack occurs when blood flow to the heart is stopped. Blood flow can be cut off by a buildup of fat and cholesterol in the blood vessels (atherosclerosis) that lead to the heart or by a clot stuck in one of the blood vessels. Part of the heart muscle dies or is damaged during a heart attack.

WARNING SIGNS

Heart Attack

- Prolonged pain, tightness, pressure, or squeezing in the chest
- Pain that spreads to the neck, shoulders, arms, or jaw
- Shortness of breath or hiccups
- Sweating
- Nausea
- Dizziness or fainting

NOTE: If you have nerve damage to your heart, you may not have pain.

If you have suffered a heart attack caused by a blockage in an artery, you may need surgery. In arterial bypass surgery, a healthy vein is taken from another part of the body and sewn onto the blocked artery above and below the blockage. Blood then flows around the blockage. In laser angioplasty, a laser beam melts the blockage. In balloon angioplasty, the narrowed part of the artery is stretched by an inflated balloon. To keep the artery open, the surgeon may insert a stint, which is like a small rigid pipe. In atherectomy, a blocked artery is opened by boring a hole through the blockage.

BRAIN

Lack of blood flow to the brain can cause a stroke. Blood flow can be cut off by a buildup of fat and cholesterol in the blood vessels (atherosclerosis) that lead to the brain. This type of stroke is an ischemic stroke. It is the most common type.

If blood flow to the brain is blocked only for a brief time, it is called a transient ischemic attack, or TIA. Your body may release enzymes that dissolve the clot quickly and restore blood flow. If you have TIAs often, you are more likely to have a major ischemic stroke.

Another type of stroke is a hemorrhagic stroke. It occurs when a blood vessel in your brain leaks or breaks. The most common cause of hemorrhagic strokes is high blood pressure.

If you have had an ischemic stroke, you may be given drugs to prevent new clots from forming or an existing clot from get-

---

WARNING SIGNS

Stroke or TIA

- You are suddenly weak or numb in your face, an arm, or a leg.
- Your sight is suddenly dim, blurred, or lost.
- You can't speak or can't understand someone else who is talking.
- You have a sudden headache.
- You feel dizzy or unsteady, or you suddenly fall.

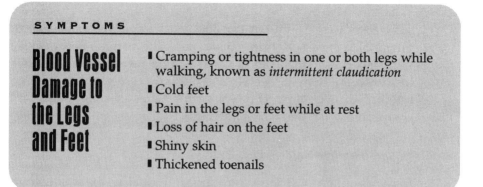

SYMPTOMS

Blood Vessel Damage to the Legs and Feet

- Cramping or tightness in one or both legs while walking, known as *intermittent claudication*
- Cold feet
- Pain in the legs or feet while at rest
- Loss of hair on the feet
- Shiny skin
- Thickened toenails

ting bigger. Occasionally, surgery (a carotid endarterectomy) is performed to remove a blockage from the carotid artery in the neck. For a hemorrhagic stroke, you may be given drugs to reduce blood pressure.

LEGS AND FEET

Damage to the blood vessels in the legs and feet can lead to poor circulation, gangrene, and amputation. Poor circulation can slow the healing of wounds and infections. It can also cause dry gangrene, which is the death of tissues. Dry gangrene can be treated by improving blood circulation to the foot. Antibiotics can be taken to prevent the area from becoming infected with bacteria. If bacterial infection sets in, you have wet gangrene. The only treatment for wet gangrene is amputation, which is the removal of the dead tissues. It might mean you lose a toe, several toes, part of a foot, the whole foot, or even a leg.

Early blood vessel disease can be treated with exercise, drugs, or arterial bypass surgery, laser angioplasty, balloon angioplasty, or atherectomy to open blocked blood vessels.

EYES

The three main eye diseases that people with diabetes can develop are retinopathy, cataracts, and glaucoma. Of the three, retinopathy is the most common.

Retinopathy

The retina is the lining at the back of the eye that senses light. Small blood vessels bring oxygen to the retina. Retinopathy damages these small blood vessels. As a result, the retina gets less oxygen than it needs, and blood vessels enlarge in an attempt to get more. The two major types of retinopathy are nonproliferative and proliferative.

Nonproliferative Retinopathy

In nonproliferative (or background) retinopathy, the small blood vessels in the retina bulge and form pouches. This weakens the blood vessels, and they may leak a bit of fluid. This leaking does not usually harm your sight. Often, the disease never gets worse.

If the disease does get worse, the weak blood vessels leak a larger amount of fluid. They also leak blood and fats. This causes the retina to swell. The swelling will usually not harm your sight, unless it occurs in the center of the retina.

The center of the retina is the macula. The macula lets you see fine details. Swelling in the macula is *macular edema*. Macular edema can blur, distort, reduce, or darken your sight.

Nonproliferative retinopathy is found in 1 of every 5 people who are diagnosed with type 2 diabetes. Most people with type 2 diabetes do not go on to develop proliferative retinopathy.

Proliferative Retinopathy

In proliferative retinopathy, the small blood vessels are so damaged that they close off. In response, many new, very small blood vessels grow in the retina. As these new blood vessels grow, they branch out to other parts of your eye.

These changes may not affect your sight. Or these changes will make you less able to see things out of the sides of your eyes. You might also find it harder to see in the dark and to adjust from light to dark.

The new blood vessels are fragile and can cause problems. They may break and bleed into the clear gel that fills the center of the eye. This is known as a *vitreous hemorrhage*. The most common signs of vitreous hemorrhage are blurring and floating spots. If not treated, vitreous hemorrhage can cause you to lose your sight.

Broken blood vessels may cause scar tissue to form on the retina. Scar tissue can wrinkle the retina and pull it out of place. A retina that has been pulled away from the back of the eye is a *detached retina*. A detached retina will cause you to see a shadow or large dark area. It can endanger your sight.

Diabetic retinopathy can be treated and cured. The best-known treatment for retinopathy is laser surgery. A laser is used to make tiny burns in the retina. This patches up leaky vessels, destroys the extra blood vessels, and discourages new fragile vessels from growing.

Macular edema also can be treated with laser surgery. In addition, low-vision aids, such as magnifying lenses (for close-up) and telescopic lenses (for distance) may be helpful.

When there is a vitreous hemorrhage or a detached retina, a vitrectomy may be needed. A vitrectomy is an operation to remove broken blood vessels and scar tissue, to stop bleeding, to replace some of the vitreous fluid within the eye with a salt solution, and, sometimes, to repair the detached retina.

SYMPTOMS

Retinopathy

- Your sight gets blurry.
- You see floating spots.
- You see a shadow or dark area.
- You can't see things on either side of you.
- You have trouble seeing at night.
- You have trouble reading.
- Straight lines do not look straight.

Usually, you can't see the early signs of damage to your retina, but your eye doctor can.

Cataract

- Your sight is hazy, fuzzy, or blurry.
- You think you need new glasses.
- Your new glasses don't help you see any better.
- You find it harder to read and do other close work.
- You blink a lot to see better.
- You feel you have a film over your eyes.
- You feel you are looking through a cloudy piece of glass, veils, or a waterfall.
- Light from the sun or a lamp seems too bright.
- At night, headlights on other cars cause more glare than before or look double or dazzling.
- Your pupil, which is usually black, looks gray, yellow, or white.
- Colors look dull.

Cataracts

A cataract clouds the eye's lens. The lens is usually clear and lies behind the iris (the colored part of your eye) and the pupil (the dark opening). The lens focuses light onto the retina. Clouding of the lens blocks light from entering. Cataracts usually start out small. Some of them never bother your sight. Others block most or all of your sight. How a cataract will affect your sight depends on three things: 1) how large it is, 2) how thick it is, and 3) where it is on the lens. Because of these three things, signs that you have a cataract may vary.

Cataracts can be treated with surgery. The clouded lens is removed and replaced with a clear, plastic lens.

Glaucoma

Glaucoma is a buildup of fluid in the eye. The fluid buildup causes increased pressure, which can damage your optic nerve. Your optic nerve tells your brain what your eye sees. Fluid can build up when the filter it normally drains out of becomes clogged. There are two kinds of glaucoma: chronic open-angle glaucoma and acute angle-closure glaucoma.

Chronic Open-Angle Glaucoma

Chronic open-angle glaucoma is the most common type. In this type, fluid pressure rises slowly over many years. You usually won't notice it. You might feel the increased pressure in your eye, or your eyes may keep tearing. As glaucoma worsens, you may notice that your sight is slightly blurry or foggy. You may feel that your glasses should be changed. You may have a hard time seeing in the dark. If not treated, you may lose your sight.

Acute Angle-Closure Glaucoma

Acute angle-closure glaucoma is the less common type. In this type, fluid pressure builds up quickly. Your eyes hurt a lot. They are blurry and keep tearing. You see colored halos around bright lights. You may even vomit. If you have any of these signs, go to a hospital emergency room right away.

Glaucoma is treated with prescription eyedrops or pills that decrease the amount of fluid the eye makes. Two other treatments are trabeculoplasty, in which a laser beam unclogs the filter, and trabeculectomy, in which the clogged filter is bypassed and a new opening is created for fluid to escape the eye.

KIDNEYS

Your kidneys clean your blood by letting wastes pass into the urine. Kidney disease, or nephropathy, is damage to the small blood vessels of the kidneys that do the cleaning.

People with type 2 diabetes are more likely to get kidney disease if they also have high blood pressure. The combination of high blood glucose levels and high blood pressure can overwork and weaken the blood vessels.

Overworked, weak blood vessels may start to leak. One thing they leak is a protein called albumin. A small amount of albumin in the urine is the first outward sign of kidney damage. As

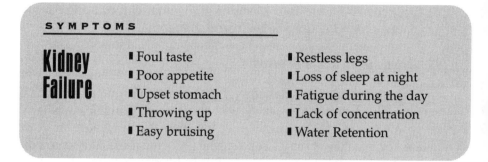

SYMPTOMS

Kidney Failure

- Foul taste
- Poor appetite
- Upset stomach
- Throwing up
- Easy bruising

- Restless legs
- Loss of sleep at night
- Fatigue during the day
- Lack of concentration
- Water Retention

more and more albumin leaks into the urine, the level of albumin in the blood falls.

One job of albumin is to hold water in the blood. If there is not enough albumin in the blood, water leaks out of the blood vessels. The water can end up in the ankles, the abdomen, and the chest. This is called edema. Water in these places may be the first physical signs that something is wrong with your kidneys.

After a time, some of the leaky blood vessels just stop working. This makes more work for the blood vessels that are still good. At first, the good blood vessels work harder to make up for the ones that have stopped. Then they, too, stop working. As more blood vessels stop, fewer are left to do the work. Eventually, none of the blood vessels are able to remove wastes. Wastes build up in the blood.

Wastes in the blood rise to toxic levels when the kidneys' blood vessels are no longer filtering. This is kidney failure or end-stage renal disease.

A person with kidney failure needs to have either a kidney transplant or dialysis. In a kidney transplant, the person gets a new kidney from someone else. In dialysis, a solution or a machine cleans the blood.

NERVES

Nerve damage, or neuropathy, is very common in people with type 2 diabetes. Neuropathy can affect any of the nerves outside your brain and spinal cord. These are peripheral nerves. There are three types of peripheral nerves: motor, sensory, and autonomic. Motor nerves control voluntary muscle movement. Sensory nerves allow you to feel and touch. Autonomic nerves control involuntary activities, like digestion. They also allow you to receive signals such as that of a full bladder, and, for men, these nerves control the ability to have an erection. There are many types of neuropathy.

Distal Symmetric Polyneuropathy

Distal symmetric polyneuropathy is nerve damage to the feet and legs and sometimes the hands. It is the most common form of neuropathy. People with this type of neuropathy may have numbness or loss of feeling; muscle weakness; tingling or prickling sensations; shooting or stabbing pain; pain on contact with bed sheets or clothing; the sensation of bugs crawling over the skin; or the sensation of walking on a strange surface.

The major goal of treatment for distal symmetric polyneuropathy is pain relief. Getting greater control of your blood glucose levels, using a TENS (transcutaneous electrical nerve stimulation) unit, using prescription topical creams, or taking prescription pills may ease your pain.

Charcot Foot or Joint

Charcot foot, also called neuropathic arthropathy, usually starts with a loss of feeling in the foot, sudden swelling, redness, and warmth. But what you may notice first is that you can't get your shoe on. If you have these symptoms, keep your weight off the foot and go to your doctor immediately. Early treatment for Charcot foot is crucial; if you continue to walk on the foot, bones in the arch and ankle will fracture and collapse. This will cause a deformed foot.

Early treatment can stop the breakdown of bone and promote healing. The foot is usually put into a cast for 3 to 4 months. This keeps the joint from moving and keeps weight off the foot. Later, as the foot heals, you can wear extra-depth or custom-molded shoes. Surgery can restore a deformed foot.

Cranial Neuropathy

Cranial neuropathy affects the nerves that control sight, eye movement, hearing, and taste. It can cause facial pain and temporary paralysis of eye muscles or parts of the face. It usually goes away without treatment.

Autonomic Neuropathy

Autonomic neuropathy can affect the nerves that control your heart, lungs, blood vessels, stomach, intestines, bladder, and sex organs.

Heart, Lungs, and Blood Vessels

Nerve damage to your heart, lungs, and blood vessels can affect your heart rate and blood pressure. Your heart may pound hard and fast even when you are at rest. You may get dizzy or feel faint when you stand up quickly. This is because your blood pressure drops. Your blood pressure may go up when you are sleeping and down when you are standing. You may have a painless heart attack.

Prescription medications can control your blood pressure. In addition, you can try to stand up slowly when you get out of bed, avoid standing for long periods, and elevate your head when you sleep.

Stomach

Nerve damage to your stomach can affect digestion by delaying the stomach's ability to empty. You may feel bloated, even after a small meal, and sick to your stomach. You may vomit food that you ate more than one meal before. Treatment may involve eating six or more small liquid meals; eating more high-fiber, low-fat foods; and taking prescription medications that stimulate the stomach to empty.

Intestines

Damage to nerves in your intestines can cause diarrhea or constipation. These conditions can be relieved by prescription or over-the-counter medications that your health care provider recommends. Drinking more water and eating more high-fiber foods may be all that is needed for constipation.

Bladder

If the nerves in your bladder are damaged, you will not be able to tell when your bladder is full of urine. You may dribble or wet yourself. The urine that stays in your bladder may cause a urinary tract infection.

Treatment of this condition usually requires that you urinate every 3 or 4 hours when you are awake, even if you feel as if you don't need to. After you urinate, press down on the lower abdomen to help empty the bladder. Other treatments include use of a catheter, prescription medications, and surgery.

Sex Organs

Nerve damage to the sex organs can cause impotence in men and vaginal dryness and loss of sensation in women. Impotence can be treated in several ways: with injections of drugs; with use of external erection aids, such as a vacuum that pulls blood into the penis; or with penis implants. In some cases, your physician may prescribe the drug Viagra®. However, if you have high or low blood pressure, have had a stroke, or have problems with

WAYS TO PREVENT COMPLICATIONS

	Blood Vessels	Heart	Brain	Legs and Feet	Eyes	Kidneys	Nerves
Control Blood Glucose	●	●	●	●	●	●	●
Quit Smoking	●	●	●	●	●		●
Control High Blood Pressure	●	●	●	●	●	●	●
Lower High Cholesterol	●	●	●	●	●		●
Exercise Regularly	●	●	●	●			
Maintain Healthy Weight	●	●	●	●			
Get Regular Checkups	●	●		●	●	●	●
Drink Less Alcohol	●	●	●	●			●
Reduce Stress	●	●	●		●	●	

your heart, kidneys, or liver, this drug will likely not be prescribed. Vaginal dryness can be treated with over-the-counter or prescription lubricants or creams.

Compression Mononeuropathy

Compression mononeuropathy is damage to a single nerve. Damage occurs when nerves are pressed against bone, cartilage, or other organs.

Carpal tunnel syndrome is the most common compression mononeuropathy. It occurs when the median nerve, which supplies feeling to the hand, is compressed at the wrist by connective tissue that has become thickened. Symptoms include numbness, swelling, or prickling in the fingers with or without pain.

Treatment for carpal tunnel syndrome includes getting greater control of your blood glucose, wearing wrist splints, taking prescribed medications, or having surgery to remove tissues squeezing the nerve. If untreated, carpal tunnel syndrome can become permanent and disabling.

BLOOD PRESSURE

People with diabetes are more likely to have high blood pressure, or hypertension, than people without diabetes. High blood pressure usually has no symptoms. The only way to know if you have high blood pressure is to get it checked. Your blood pressure should be checked each time you visit your diabetes care provider.

How Is Your Blood Pressure?	
	Blood Pressure Reading (in mmHg)
Normal blood pressure	Less than 130/85
High-normal blood pressure	130/85 to 139/89
Mild hypertension	140/90 to 159/99
Moderate hypertension	160/100 to 179/109
Severe hypertension	180/110 to 209/119
Very severe hypertension	More than 210/120

Blood pressure is reported as two numbers. The first number is the systolic pressure. Systolic pressure is the force of your blood when your heart contracts. The second number is the diastolic pressure. Diastolic pressure is the force of your blood when your heart relaxes.

A reading of "120 over 80" means a systolic pressure of 120 and a diastolic pressure of 80. It is written as 120/80 mmHg (millimeters [mm] of mercury [Hg]).

If you find out that your blood pressure is high, you and your health care team can take steps to control it. Your health care team will first try to find out the cause of your high blood pressure.

Sometimes, there is a specific cause, such as a kidney problem, hormone disorder, pregnancy, or the use of birth control pills. When high blood pressure is linked to a specific cause, it is called secondary hypertension. If you have secondary hypertension, your health care provider will treat the cause first.

Most of the time, there is no obvious cause for high blood pressure. When there is no obvious cause, it is called essential hypertension. If you have essential hypertension, there are things you can do to bring your blood pressure down without taking drugs.

Many people can lower their blood pressure by losing weight through diet and exercise. Some people can lower blood pressure by cutting salt in their diet or avoiding alcohol. Other times, blood pressure drugs are needed.

Blood pressure drugs used most often in people with diabetes are ACE (angiotensin-converting enzyme) inhibitors, alpha$_1$-receptor blockers, calcium antagonists, and thiazide diuretics in small doses.

These blood pressure drugs do not raise blood glucose levels, but they all have side effects. Ask your diabetes care provider or pharmacist about them.

BLOOD FATS

Blood fats include cholesterol and triglycerides. People with diabetes often have high blood fat levels. Find out what your blood fat levels are.

Have your blood fat levels tested at least once a year, or more often if your diabetes care provider recommends. If you find that your blood fat levels are high, try the following steps to lower them:

- Control your diabetes.
- Lose weight if you need to.
- Cut back on fat in your diet.
- Replace saturated fats with unsaturated fats.
- Eat fewer foods high in cholesterol.
- Eat more foods high in fiber.
- Exercise regularly.
- Quit smoking.

BLOOD FATS (LIPID) PROFILE (IN MG/DL)			
	Desirable	Borderline	High
LDL Cholesterol	Under 100	100–129	130 or above
HDL Cholesterol	Under 45	35–45	35 or above
Triglycerides	Under 200	200–399	400 or above

Coping With Complications

If you have a complication, learn all you can about it. The more you know about your complication, the more in control you will feel.

Talk with family and friends. Tell them what's going on and what they can do to help.

Seek counseling. If you find it hard to talk with family and friends, you may want to get counseling from a social worker or psychologist.

Join a support group. Other people who have your complications can give you moral support. And you may get new ideas on treatment options or specialists. Your diabetes care provider or local American Diabetes Association affiliate or chapter may be able to help you find a support group.

See a specialist. Think about going to a specialist who deals with your complication. Your own diabetes care provider may be able to refer you to one.

Ask questions about treatments. What are the treatments? What are the side effects of the treatments? How much do these treatments cost? How often will I need treatments? Will I need new drugs after the treatment? How many patients with this problem have you treated? What has happened to those patients?

Try to get a second opinion. Check your health insurance. It might cover a second opinion.

Look for organizations that focus on your complication. Organizations like the National Kidney Foundation, the American Foundation for the Blind, and the National Amputation Foundation have programs and services. For more information on these and other organizations, see RESOURCES at the end of this book.

Think positive. Thinking good thoughts about yourself and about things in your life can make your life happier, maybe even longer. Thinking too much about things you don't like or that frighten you can only make living with complications harder for you and your loved ones.

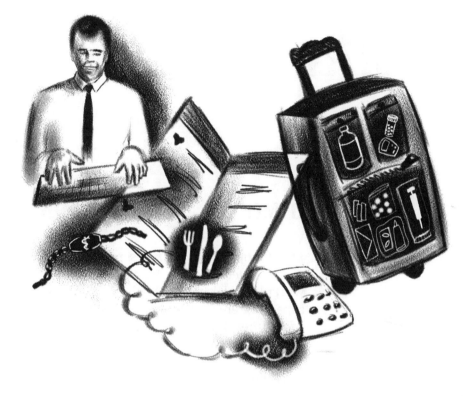

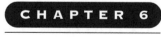

CHAPTER 6

LIFESTYLE

LIFESTYLE

EMPLOYMENT

People with diabetes may be discriminated against (treated unfairly) in the workplace. Discrimination can occur in any aspect of employment, including application procedures, hiring, training, pay, benefits, promotions, tenure, leaves of absence, layoffs, and firings.

Whether you are looking for a job, waiting for a promotion, or deciding whether to tell your employer that you have been diagnosed with diabetes, the first step to getting fair treatment is to know your rights.

You don't have to tell a potential employer that you have diabetes. But if you decide to talk about your diabetes during an interview, emphasize the positive. Refer to any awards you've won in previous jobs or other examples of your hard work and good skills. If you haven't used much sick leave, point that out, too.

A potential employer cannot ask you about your health or make you get a physical exam before offering you a job. However, some jobs require all employees to get a physical exam after they are hired.

If you have to get an employment physical exam, don't change your treatment plan right before the exam. Changes in routine can affect your diabetes control. Be aware that the company's doctor is probably not a specialist in diabetes care. You may want to point out the steps you take to maintain control of your diabetes. For some jobs, you may be required to show that you have good blood glucose control and to set up a plan for keeping that control on the job.

The employer is allowed to take back a job offer because of the results of a medical exam—but only if the reason is related to the job.

If you are not required to tell your employer about your diabetes as part of a medical exam or licensing process, then whether or not you tell is completely up to you. But there are some advantages to telling your employer and/or your coworkers. Being open about your diabetes can show others that people with diabetes are safe and responsible workers. If you take insulin, it may help you if your coworkers know how to recognize, and perhaps treat, low blood glucose. Also, if you need to make changes in your work schedule because of your diabetes, your employer may be more understanding of your needs.

Another important reason to tell people is that this is the only way your employment rights will be protected by the Americans with Disabilities Act of 1990. The Americans with Disabilities Act is a civil rights law that protects the employment rights of people with diabetes who are considered disabled. You are considered disabled if one of these statements is true:

1. Diabetes greatly limits one or more of your major life activities. Some major life activities include, but are not limited to, seeing, hearing, speaking, walking, breathing, doing manual tasks, learning, caring for yourself, and working.
2. You have a record of a disability because at one time, diabetes greatly limited one or more of your major life activities.
3. Your employer regards you as disabled because you have diabetes. It does not matter how your diabetes has actually affected you.

Under this law, your employer cannot discriminate against you if you are qualified for the job and if you can do the job with or without "reasonable accommodation." Accommodation means that your employer makes changes in your work, work area, or schedule or provides equipment or training to help you do the job. The employer is required to make accommodation unless it would cause an "undue hardship" because it is very difficult or expensive to do.

Employers do not have to give you more sick leave than other workers. However, under the Family and Medical Leave Act you may be entitled to 12 weeks of unpaid leave per year to deal with your own or a close family member's diabetes care. This leave can be taken in small blocks of time.

In addition, employers do not have to give you preference over other equally qualified people who apply for the job. They can choose whoever they feel can best perform a job. However, an employer will run into problems if he or she hires someone less qualified, while refusing employment to a more qualified person who happens to have diabetes.

If you are rejected for a position, ask for a written explanation. Keep copies of the job announcement and your job application. Make notes of your conversations and meetings with potential employers, including dates, times, places, names of those present, and the subjects discussed.

The Americans with Disabilities Act applies to private companies, state and local governments, employment agencies, and labor unions. The Act does not apply to employers with fewer than 15 workers, Native American tribes, tax-exempt private clubs, and the federal government. People who work for the federal government or for organizations that get federal funds are protected by the Federal Rehabilitation Act of 1973. In addition, all states have their own employment rights laws. Some of these laws provide even more protection than the federal laws.

Job discrimination can be hard to prove. If you think an employer has discriminated against you because of diabetes, follow these steps:

• Try solving the problem by talking directly with the employer.
• Get the help of a union or employee group.
• Talk to a lawyer. With a telephone call or letter, a lawyer may

be able to resolve the problem quickly, making a lawsuit unnecessary.

- File charges with the Equal Employment Opportunity Commission (EEOC), your state anti-discrimination agency, or for federal workers, your agency's Equal Employment Opportunity Office. You must file a charge before going to court and the time limits to do so are very short. You can reach the EEOC at 1-800-669-4000.
- If you are asked to leave your job, look for other work. If your case goes to court, the court may want to see that you can and want to work.

If you win your case, the employer usually must place you in the position you would have had, give you back pay (the sum of wages that you've lost) and other damages, and pay your costs and lawyers fees. For more information, contact the American Diabetes Association at 1-800-DIABETES (342-2383) and request the ADA's packet on Employment Discrimination.

TRAVEL

At some time you will likely want or need to take a trip. You can go anywhere you want to go. It just takes a little planning to handle your diabetes. How you prepare will depend on where you are going and for how long. It is important to plan ahead.

Planning Ahead

- Before a long trip, get a medical exam to be sure all is well.
- Get any shots—if you need them—at least 1 month before you leave.
- Get a letter from your diabetes care provider saying that you have diabetes. Be sure the letter lists any medications, such as diabetes pills or insulin, that you take or devices, such as a blood glucose meter or syringes, that you use. It should also point out any allergies or adverse reactions to food and medications you may have. This letter will save you a lot of trouble when you go through customs and make things easier if you get ill while you are traveling.

- Get a prescription from your health care provider for insulin or diabetes pills. Even if you don't need a prescription in your state, you may need one in other states or foreign countries. Be prepared so you'll always be able to get insulin, syringes, or diabetes pills if you need them.
- If you're traveling in the United States, take along a list of American Diabetes Association affiliates (see RESOURCES). They can refer you to health care providers in the area.
- If you're really in trouble, you can always go to an emergency room at a hospital or to an urgent care or quick care center in the United States.
- If you're going overseas, write for a list of International Diabetes Federation groups (see RESOURCES). You may also want to request a list of English-speaking foreign health care providers (see RESOURCES). If an emergency occurs while you're traveling and you don't have such a list, contact the American Consulate, American Express, or local medical schools for a list of health care providers.
- Wear a medical I.D. (identification) bracelet or necklace that indicates that you have diabetes.
- If you're leaving the country, try to learn how to say "I have diabetes" and "Sugar or orange juice, please," in the languages of the areas you will be visiting. Write the phrases down to carry with you. You can point to them if you have trouble pronouncing them.

What to Pack

Pack twice as much medication and blood-testing supplies as you think you'll need, because it's always better to have more than not enough. Pack half in a bag that you'll keep with you at all times. Other stuff to pack in this bag includes:

- The letter from your diabetes care provider stating that you have diabetes
- Prescriptions for diabetes pills, insulin, and other medications
- Diabetes pills
- Insulin

- Syringes, jet injectors, insulin pens, or pump
- Other medications
- Glucose meter
- Test strips
- Lancets
- Alcohol (if used)
- Cotton or tissues
- Spare batteries for glucose meter
- Glucagon kit
- Glucose tablets or gel
- Snacks, such as cheese and crackers, juice, and fruit

Traveling With Insulin

Pack insulin in bags that protect it from extreme heat or cold. For example, if you are traveling by car in the summer, keep insulin in an insulated container with ice in a bag or "blue ice" (but don't allow the insulin to freeze), a cool damp cloth, or some other cooling agent. Your automobile glove compartment and trunk can get awfully hot. Backpacks and cycle bags also can get quite hot in direct sunlight.

If you are flying and crossing over time zones, here is a rule of thumb: eastward travel results in a shorter day; thus, if you inject insulin, less insulin may be needed. On the other hand, traveling west gives you a longer day and may require more insulin. If you have concerns about insulin adjustment while crossing time zones, take your round-trip airline flight schedule to your diabetes care provider along with information on the time zone changes. Work out the appropriate adjustments in intermediate- or long-acting and short-acting insulins for travel days. These may depend on your meal schedule and plans for sleep or activity on arrival at your destination. Self-monitoring of blood glucose while traveling will help you make informed decisions.

Insulins sold abroad may differ from the U-100 used in the United States. If you buy insulin overseas, it may be a different strength (U-40 or U-80). You'll need to buy syringes to match the insulin to avoid getting the wrong dose. If you use U-100 syringes for U-40 insulin, you will be taking much less insulin than was prescribed. If you use U-100 insulin in a U-80 syringe, you will be taking too much insulin. Match the syringe to the insulin.

EATING OUT

Today, more and more people eat out at restaurants. Restaurant owners have become more health-conscious. Most restaurant menus now feature "lite" or "healthy" entrees. All eating places offer sugar substitutes and diet beverages. Most serve fruit juice and decaffeinated coffee. Some have reduced-calorie salad dressings, low-fat or skim milk, and salt substitutes. It's also easy to find salads, fish and seafood, vegetables, baked or broiled food, and whole-grain breads.

More restaurants are offering menus that list calories and nutrients or provide the information on request. If you ask, chefs can sometimes create low-fat entrees just for you. Some cooks will remove the skin from a chicken, omit extra butter on the dish, broil instead of fry, and serve sauces on the side. There are restaurants that will allow you to order small portions at reduced prices. All these improvements make it easier to fit restaurant foods into your meal plan.

Ask your dietitian or health care provider about eating out. Find out which part of your meal plan is most important to follow. For some people, cutting calories is most important, but for others, it may be avoiding fat and eating high-fiber foods. Try to follow your meal plan as much as possible. Here are some suggestions.

Table Tips

- If you can, pick a restaurant that offers a wide variety of choices.
- If you don't know the ingredients in a dish or the serving size, ask.
- Try to eat the same size servings that you eat at home. If the servings are too large, use a doggie bag before you start eating, or share portions with your dining partner.
- Eat slowly. Take the time to savor each bite.

- Ask that fish or meat be broiled with little added fat.
- Ask that sour cream or butter for the baked potato be put on the side or left off.
- If you are on a low-sodium diet or are just trying to cut back, ask that no salt or as little as possible be added to your food.
- Ask that sauces, gravy, and dressings be served on the side.
- Avoid breaded or fried foods. If the food arrives breaded, you can peel off the outer coating or send it back if you specifically ordered it without breading.
- Use the menu creatively. For instance, order the fruit cup appetizer or the breakfast melon for your dinner dessert.
- Ask for substitutions, such as low-fat cottage cheese, baked potato, or even a double portion of a vegetable instead of French fries.
- Ask about low-calorie items, like salad dressings, even if they're not listed on the menu.
- Substitute low-calorie or calorie-free beverages for alcoholic beverages.

It may help to phone ahead. When you make the reservation, it's possible to ask, for example, that your food be prepared with vegetable oil and little salt and be broiled instead of fried. Remember, you are the customer; you are the one paying the bill. It is okay to ask for what you need.

If you like the healthy choices on a restaurant's menu, let the manager know. If you'd like to see more low-calorie, low-cholesterol choices on the menu, say so. Restaurants, like any business, only know what you want if you tell them.

Eating on Time

If you take diabetes pills or insulin, ordering the right foods isn't your only concern. You need to think about when you eat as well. Eating around the same times each day helps keep your blood glucose levels more even.

- If you're eating with others, ask if they would mind eating at your usual time.

MAKING HEALTHY CHOICES WHEN EATING OUT

	Choose	Avoid
Appetizers	Tomato juice, unsweetened juice Clear broth, bouillon, consommé Raw vegetables Fresh fruit, unsweetened Fresh steamed seafood	Sweetened juices Cream soups, thick soups Marinated vegetables Canned fruit cocktail Breaded or fried seafood
Eggs	Poached or boiled	Fried, creamed, or scrambled
Salads	Tossed vegetable Cottage cheese	Coleslaw Canned fruit or gelatin salads
Breads	Whole-grain rolls, crackers, biscuits, breads	Sweet rolls, coffee cake, croissants
Potatoes, Pasta, Rice	Baked, boiled, or steamed potatoes Steamed rice or pasta	Fried, French fried, creamed, scalloped, or au gratin potatoes
Fats	Low-calorie salad dressing Low-fat sour cream or yogurt	Regular salad dressing Regular sour cream Gravy, cream sauces
Vegetables	Raw, stewed, steamed, or boiled	Creamed, scalloped, or au gratin
Meat, Poultry, and Fish	Roasted, baked, or broiled Lean meats with skin or fat removed	Fried, battered, or breaded Cured meats, organ meats Stews and casseroles Gravy, cream sauces
Desserts	Fresh fruit or fruit juice Nonfat or low-fat frozen yogurt	Sweetened fruit Pudding, custard, pastries
Beverages	Coffee, tea (decaffeinated) Skim milk Diet soda Water	Chocolate milk, cocoa Milk shakes Regular soft drinks

- Try to avoid the busiest hours at the restaurant so you are less likely to have to wait.
- Ask whether special requests will take extra time to be prepared and served.
- If your meal is going to be later than usual, eat a piece of fruit or bread at your usual mealtime.
- If dinner will be very late, eat your bedtime snack before dinner.

Fast Food

Today's fast-food restaurants are offering healthier choices—such as salads, baked potatoes, chili, and grilled chicken—that make it easier to fit fast food into a healthy eating plan. But there are still plenty of high-fat, high-calorie fast-food choices out there. Be careful what you order. It is possible to eat an entire day's worth of fat, salt, and calories in just one fast-food meal.

Follow the guidelines your dietitian or health care provider has given you. You may be counting calories, grams of carbohydrate, or grams of fat. If you have not been given guidelines, try to keep these general rules in mind: 1) eat a variety of foods in moderate amounts, 2) limit your fat intake, and 3) watch the amount of sodium in your food choices.

Many fast-food restaurants can give you the nutritional information on their food if you ask. By knowing the nutritional value of fast-food items, you can choose foods that will fit into your meal plan. If you have fast food for one meal, try to eat low-fat foods, like fruits and vegetables, for your other meals that day. Here are some tips to help you choose well:

- For breakfast, try a plain bagel, toast, or English muffin. Drink fruit juice or low-fat milk. Order cold cereal with skim milk, pancakes without butter, or plain scrambled eggs. Avoid bacon and sausage.
- Load up on lettuce and vegetables at a salad bar. Go easy on the dressing, bacon bits, cheeses, croutons, mayonnaise, and macaroni salads. Too much of even a low-calorie salad dressing can make a difference. Check the number of calories on the packet.
- Order regular or junior-size sandwiches rather than the larger "jumbo," "giant," or "deluxe" sandwiches to get fewer calories and less fat, cholesterol, and sodium.
- Choose plain lean roast beef, turkey or chicken breast, or lean ham sandwiches.
- Skip the croissant and eat your sandwich on a bun or bread instead to save calories and fat.
- Choose chicken or fish if it is roasted, unbreaded, grilled, baked, or broiled without fat. Chicken or fish that is battered, breaded, or fried is higher in calories and fat than a hamburger.

- Stay away from double burgers or super hot dogs with cheese, chili, or sauces. Cheese can carry an extra 100 calories, as well as extra fat and sodium.
- Order items plain without toppings, rich sauces, or mayonnaise. Add lettuce, tomato, onion, and mustard instead.
- Choose cheese pizza with vegetables. Other toppings, such as pepperoni, sausage, and extra cheese, add calories, fat, and sodium. **A word of caution**: The high carbohydrate content of pizza can make blood glucose levels go really high in some people. The high fat content of pizza may delay the blood glucose rise until several hours later. Check your blood glucose at different times after eating pizza to learn how it affects you.
- Order tacos, tostados, bean burritos, soft tacos, and other non-fried items when eating Mexican fast foods. Choose chicken over beef. Avoid beans refried in lard. Pile on extra lettuce, tomatoes, and salsa. Go easy on cheese, sour cream, and guacamole. Watch out for the deep-fried taco salad shell—a taco salad can have more than 1,000 calories!
- If you have room for dessert, go for sugar-free nonfat frozen yogurt. Ices, sorbets, and sherbets have less fat and fewer calories than ice cream. But they are full of sugar and can send your blood glucose too high unless you work the extra sugar into your meal plan. Some places now offer fresh fruit!

Eating out can be one of life's great pleasures. By making the right choices and balancing the meals you eat out with the meals you eat at home, you can enjoy yourself and take care of your diabetes at the same time.

ALCOHOL, DRUGS, AND TOBACCO

Alcohol

One or two drinks a day will have little effect on your blood glucose level if you have good control of your diabetes, are free of complications, and drink the alcohol close to or with a meal. But drinking two drinks on an empty stomach can cause low blood glucose if you are taking diabetes pills or insulin or if you were just exercising or about to exercise.

Usually, if your blood glucose drops too low, your liver puts more glucose into the blood. (The liver has its own supply of glucose, called glycogen.) But when alcohol, a toxin, is in the body, the liver wants to get rid of it first. While the liver is taking care of the alcohol, it may let blood glucose drop to dangerous levels.

To avoid low blood glucose, always have something to eat when you have a drink. Check your blood glucose before, during, and after drinking. Alcohol can lower blood glucose as long as 8 to 12 hours after your last drink.

Alcohol on the breath may mislead people into thinking you are drunk, and you may not get the treatment you need for low blood glucose. If you drink and then drive when you have low blood glucose, you may be pulled over for drunk driving. When you drink, let someone else drive.

If you treat your diabetes with diet and exercise, low blood glucose when drinking is less likely to happen. Still, alcohol can disrupt your meal plan.

Work with a dietitian to include your favorite drink in your meal plan. Be aware that regular beer, sweet wines, and wine coolers will raise your blood glucose more than light beer, dry wines, and liquors (such as vodka, scotch, and whiskey) because they contain more carbohydrate. Carbohydrate is the nutrient that raises blood glucose the most.

Alcoholic beverages supply lots of calories (anywhere from 60 to 300 calories each) but few nutrients. You'll need to add the calories from alcoholic drinks to your daily calorie count.

To cut calories
- Use 80 proof in place of 100 proof alcohol. The lower the proof number, the less alcohol in the liquor. Each gram of alcohol has 7 calories.
- Put less liquor in your drink.
- Use no-calorie mixers, such as diet sodas, club soda, or water.
- Choose light beer over regular beer.
- Choose dry wine over sweet or fruity wines and wine coolers.
- Try a wine spritzer made with a small amount of wine and a lot of club soda.

Beverage	Serving (ounces)	Alcohol (g)	Carbohydrates (g)	Calories	Exchanges
Beer					
Regular	12	13	13	150	1 Carbohydrate, 2 Fat
Light	12	11	5	100	2 Fat
Distilled spirits, 80 proof (gin, rum, vodka, whiskey, scotch)	1½	14	Trace	100	2 Fat
Dry brandy, cognac	1	11	Trace	75	1½ Fat
Table wine					
Dry white	4	11	Trace	80	2 Fat
Red or rose	4	12	2	85	2 Fat
Sweet wine	4	12	5	105	½ Carbohydrate, 2 Fat
Light wine	4	6	1	50	1 Fat
Wine cooler	12	13	30	215	2 Carbohydrate, 2 Fat
Nonalcoholic wines	4	Trace	6–7	25–35	½ Carbohydrate
Sparkling wines					
Champagne	4	12	4	100	2 Fat
Sweet kosher wine	4	12	12	132	1 Carbohydrate, 2 Fat
Appetizer/ dessert wines					
Sherry	2	9	2	74	1½ Fat
Sweet sherry, port, muscatel	2	9	7	90	½ Carbohydrate, 1½ Fat
Cordials, liqueurs	1½	13	18	160	1 Carbohydrate, 2 Fat
Vermouth					
Dry	3	13	4	105	2 Fat
Sweet	3	13	14	140	1 Carbohydrate, 2 Fat
Cocktails					
Bloody Mary	5	14	5	116	1 Vegetable, 2 Fat
Daiquiri	2	14	2	111	2 Fat
Manhattan	2	17	2	178	2½ Fat
Martini	2½	22	Trace	156	3½ Fat
Old Fashioned	4	26	Trace	180	4 Fat
Tom Collins	7½	16	3	120	2½ Fat
Mixes					
Mineral water	Any	0	0	0	Free
Sugar-free tonic	Any	0	0	0	Free
Club soda	Any	0	0	0	Free
Diet soda	Any	0	0	0	Free
Tomato juice	4	0	5	25	1 Vegetable
Bloody Mary	4	0	5	25	1 Vegetable
Orange juice	4	0	15	60	1 Fruit
Grapefruit juice	4	0	15	60	1 Fruit
Pineapple juice	4	0	15	60	1 Fruit

Cooking with Alcohol

When alcohol is heated in cooking, either on top of the stove or in the oven, some of it evaporates. How much of it evaporates depends on how long you cook it. If you cook it for 30 minutes or less, about one-third of the alcohol calories will remain. You'll need to count them in your meal plan. If you use alcohol regularly (3 times a week) in your cooking, the calories can add up.

Drugs

Certain drugs raise your blood glucose, others lower it. Learning how drugs affect your diabetes control will help you avoid problems.

Marijuana

Marijuana increases your appetite, making it more difficult to keep to your meal plan. If you give in to eating more, your blood glucose may rise too high.

Cocaine

Cocaine reduces your appetite. But because it acts like adrenaline, it may raise your blood glucose level. It can raise blood pressure or cause sudden heart attacks. Heavy use leads to atherosclerosis, and the risk for this disease is already high for people with diabetes.

Caffeine

Caffeine is found in coffee, tea, chocolate, and many soft drinks. It could raise your blood glucose level a small amount. Other side effects include not being able to sleep, shaking, and increased blood pressure and heart rate. You could confuse your reaction to caffeine with the symptoms of low blood glucose.

Tobacco

Smoking or chewing tobacco is especially dangerous for people with diabetes. Smoking increases your risk of having heart disease and blood vessel disease. Chewing tobacco increases your risk for oral cancer.

Here are a few suggestions that might help you quit smoking, courtesy of the National Cancer Institute:

- Switch to a brand you don't like.
- Buy cigarettes lower in tar and nicotine.
- Put your packs in a zippered pocket or purse compartment so they won't be so easy to reach for.
- List all the reasons why quitting is a good idea.
- Set a quitting date, then work toward it.
- Each day, decide how many cigarettes you will smoke.
- Postpone your first cigarette for an hour or two, and try smoking only half a cigarette.
- Find a healthy habit, such as a quick walk after a meal, to replace smoking.
- Don't put yourself into situations where you "usually" smoke until your resolve is strong.
- Talk to your health care provider about aids to help you stop smoking.

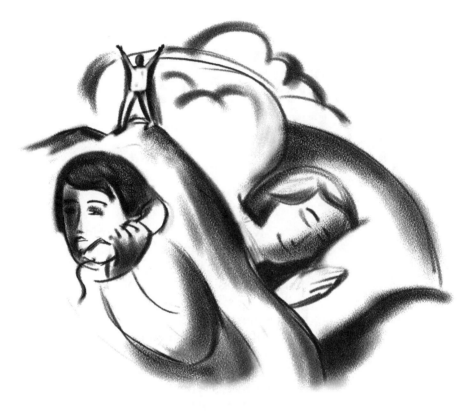

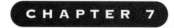

CHAPTER 7

MAINTAINING YOUR MENTAL HEALTH

MAINTAINING YOUR MENTAL HEALTH

Living with diabetes can bring on many powerful emotions: denial (I don't believe this is happening to me), anger (why me?), depression (I feel sad and hopeless), guilt (I must have done something wrong), helplessness (I can't cope with this), or lowered self-esteem (something must be wrong with me).

These feelings are normal. They can be part of the process you go through before you accept diabetes. Accepting diabetes means that you take responsibility for managing it, staying in good health, and living a full life. Even after you have accepted diabetes, these feelings will never leave you completely. But you can learn how to deal with them.

DENIAL

Almost everybody goes through denial when they are first diagnosed with diabetes. The trouble comes if you keep on denying your diabetes. Continued denial keeps you from learning what you need to know to stay healthy.

Are You in Denial?

If you hear yourself thinking or saying some of these words, you may be denying some part of your diabetes care:

- One bite won't hurt.
- This sore will heal by itself.
- I'll go to the doctor later.
- I don't have time to do it.
- My diabetes isn't serious.

How to Break Away From Denial

- Ask your diabetes care provider about things you can do to care for your diabetes.
- Tell your friends and family how they can help you take care of your diabetes.
- Talk with a mental health professional. He or she can help you overcome denial.

ANGER

Diabetes and anger often go hand in hand. You may be angry that diabetes has threatened your health and disrupted your life. You may be angry at the things you now have to do to keep your diabetes in control. What fuels your anger is less important than what you do with your anger. If you don't control your anger, it will control you.

How to Control Your Anger

Learn more about it. Start an anger diary. Write down when you felt angry, where you were, who you were with, why you felt angry, and what you did. After a few weeks, read it over. Try to understand what is making you angry. The better you understand your anger, the better you will be able to control it.

Defuse it. If you feel yourself getting angry, talk slowly, take deep breaths, get a drink of water, sit down, lean back, keep your hands down at your sides.

Let it out. Do a physical activity like jogging or raking leaves. Cry over a sad movie. Write down on a piece of paper what you feel like saying or shouting. Go off by yourself and say all you want to say. Vent your anger, calm down, and then return to the situation.

Make it trivial. Ask yourself just how important it is. Some things are just too trivial to be worth your anger.

Laugh at it. Find something funny about it. Sometimes laughter can push out anger.

Let it give you strength. How you use the energy of your anger is up to you. Plan to use your anger in a way that helps you next time. Anger can give you the courage to speak up for yourself or protect someone else.

DEPRESSION

Having diabetes can be depressing. You may feel alone or set apart from your friends and family because of the extra work you do to care for your diabetes. Perhaps you are saddened by the news that you have a complication of diabetes. Maybe you're down because you've been having trouble keeping your blood glucose level where you want it to be. Feeling down once in awhile is normal. But feeling really sad and hopeless for 2 weeks or more might be a sign of serious depression.

Are You Depressed?

- Are things that used to be fun no longer fun?
- Do you have trouble falling asleep, wake up often in the night, or want to sleep a lot more than usual?
- Do you wake up earlier than usual and have trouble falling back to sleep?
- Do you eat more or less than you used to, making you gain or lose weight?
- Do you have trouble paying attention or get distracted easily?
- Do you feel drained of energy?
- Do you often feel nervous or "antsy"?
- Are you less interested in sex?
- Do you cry more often?

- Do you feel you never do anything right or think that you are a burden to other people?
- Do you feel sad or worse in the morning than you do the rest of the day?
- Do you think you would be better off dead? Do you think about hurting yourself or committing suicide?

If you answered yes to three or more of these questions, or if you answered yes to one or two questions and you have felt this way for 2 weeks or more, you may be depressed. Get help. If you answered yes to the last question, get help right away.

Help for Depression

Depression can be caused by a physical illness. Check with your health care provider to see if there is a physical cause for your depression. If a physical cause is ruled out, you may want to see a mental health professional. This person may be a psychiatrist, psychologist, psychiatric social worker, or counselor. Treatment may involve counseling or antidepressant medication or both.

GUILT

We can feel guilty for things we do and for things we don't do. If you have ever gone on an eating binge, quit an exercise program almost as soon as you started it, or neglected your blood glucose testing for a long time, you are probably well aware of how guilt can get tangled up in diabetes care.

Guilt may prompt you to get back on track and make some positive changes. But guilt is harmful when it makes you criticize yourself too much. When this happens, your self-confidence slips, and you give up on trying to do anything. Give yourself permission to slack off sometimes and to charge ahead at other times. You must respect your own energy as well as your goals.

How to Steer Away From Guilt

Make changes one at a time. Focus on one area of change at a time. For instance, don't begin a new job, start a diet, and go on an exercise program all in the same week.

Make changes gradually. Divide large changes into small steps. For example, don't expect to start a walking program by walking 45 minutes each day. Begin by walking for 10 to 15 minutes every other day. Then gradually increase your walking.

Give yourself permission to slack off sometimes. You cannot expect to follow your diabetes care plan every hour of every day. It's impossible to keep up that level of energy.

Give yourself credit for trying. It's impossible to be perfect. You will make mistakes. But what counts is that you try your best as often as you can.

Take stock of your successes. We are quick to criticize ourselves when we make a mistake. And many times we overlook our successes. For instance, you may not have worked on your exercise program for 6 months, but you have pretty much followed the pyramid in choosing foods to eat. So give yourself a pat on the back for sticking to your meal plan.

View setbacks as opportunities. Setbacks only come to those who are trying to accomplish something in the first place. Use setbacks as an opportunity to reevaluate your goals. Are these goals realistic for you right now? Are there better ways of approaching these goals?

HELPLESSNESS

Some people accept no responsibility for managing their own illness. These people have a "can't do" attitude. They are extremely dependent on family and health care providers to manage their disease for them. These people may feel that the health care provider should make all of the decisions and that all they need to do is follow "doctor's orders."

Other people think of themselves as victims. They use being a victim to get others to do what they want. Although they feel some personal responsibility, they don't look for solutions within themselves. Instead, they get angry or blame others (family, job, health care provider, or medication) when things aren't going well. And, although they complain a lot, these people make no effort to change things.

Other people look for someone else to share the blame with. They may find themselves saying, "I really eat too much and should lose 20 pounds, but my wife always cooks fried foods." By finding faults in others, these people keep themselves from examining their own role. They need to take a good look at what they see as roadblocks and come up with constructive solutions. For example, "I'll help my wife find recipes to prepare my favorite foods without frying." Now he's taking responsibility for his own life.

Once they have increased their responsibility to this level, people might hear themselves saying, "I need to lose weight, and I know it's up to me. I just haven't done it." Or, "I've been letting my control slip, and I need to improve."

Taking Responsibility for Your Diabetes

- Set a reasonable goal.
- Self-monitor your progress toward your goal.
- Ask for and receive feedback about your progress from health care providers, family, and others close to you.
- Find constructive solutions to problems that come up; don't stop at just naming the problem.
- Feel free to revise your goal to make it fit your lifestyle.
- Reward yourself for success. Let friends and family members celebrate with you, too.

When you are responsible for your diabetes care, you'll say things like, "Since I developed diabetes, I have a new way of understanding how my body uses food." Or, "Diabetes has helped me realize how much I value feeling well."

SELF-ESTEEM

Self-esteem has a strong impact on every part of your life. You do better in your work, studies, and personal relationships when you feel good about yourself. You are more likely to go after—and get—what you want out of life when you have a strong sense of your own worth. Others are more likely to think well of you, too.

Learning to Assert Yourself

Taking responsibility for your diabetes requires you to be organized and assertive. Some people find it difficult to talk about what they need. They may be embarrassed to be different or to have their needs conflict with those of the people around them. Some simply find it difficult to call attention to themselves. Others fear the imagined consequences of speaking up for themselves. Getting what you need for your diabetes is your challenge in social situations, in any relationship, in the workplace, and in the health care provider's office. Being honest about what you need can improve your care. When you are direct and honest, you give the people around you choices about how to help you. Try these basic assertiveness skills:

Learn to say "no." A simple "no, thank you" says that you respect yourself enough to act in your own best self-interest. You also respect the other person enough to know that he or she will understand.

Be firm. Decide what you need. Then find a way to get what you need or do what you need to do. Don't risk low blood glucose by waiting to eat because no one else is eating.

Be considerate. Some people may be uncomfortable when you take a blood sample for testing or inject insulin. Give your companions a choice about watching you do these tasks.

Maintain self-respect. If you respect yourself, you will have no difficulty explaining your situation ahead of time and asking for help when you need it.

Be direct. Explain things simply to others.

The way your parents, family, teachers, and friends treat you from the time you are very young colors your sense of yourself. From their treatment of you, you form a sense of who you are and whether you like yourself. But self-esteem is not fixed. It changes as you grow and accomplish new skills. In fact, it changes from day to day. You may feel better or worse about yourself depending on things like

- How you think you look that day.
- How others respond to you.
- Your physical well-being.
- How prepared you are for the day's work.
- Whether you feel hopeful or hopeless about the future.

Your self-image may suffer when you have diabetes. You may see yourself as ill or dependent. You may think less of yourself or wonder if there is something wrong with you.

Having diabetes can change your self-esteem in positive ways, too. The challenges that you meet and the decisions that you learn to make will add to your self-confidence and sense of accomplishment. Your self-esteem will bloom when you discover all the new abilities you didn't know you had. The only thing stopping you from having high self-esteem is your own belief about yourself.

How to Improve Your Self-Esteem

- Identify what would make you feel better about yourself.
- Consider ways you could make those things happen.
- Identify something you like about yourself each day. You might like the way you dress, the handiwork you do, the way you cook, the volunteer work you do, or the sports you play.
- Associate with people who are supportive and caring about you.
- Confront people who constantly criticize you. Let them know you won't tolerate it anymore.
- Tell people directly what you want and what you need rather than hoping they will pick up on nonverbal signals.
- Compliment yourself each day.
- Compliment others. They may return the favor.
- Try to have a few enjoyable moments for yourself each day.
- If none of these work, consider talking to a mental health professional.

STRESS

Stress is a part of life. Traffic jams, deadlines, relationships at home and at work, finances, injuries, or an illness, like diabetes, can all cause stress.

What Causes You to Feel Stressed?

Each one of us is different. What causes little or no stress for you may cause great stress for somebody else. Make a list of the people or things that stress you.

How Do You React to Stress?

Pay attention to how you react. How you react may be different from how someone else reacts. You may react by feeling tense, anxious, upset, or angry. You may react by feeling tired, sad, or empty. Your stomach, head, or back may hurt.

Some people react by laughing nervously or being self-critical. Others become easily discouraged or frustrated or bored. Some cry easily.

How Do You Handle Stress?

How you handle each stressful situation determines how much stress you feel. You can handle stress in a way that makes you feel in control. Or you can handle stress in a way that makes you feel worse.

Sometimes, people choose to handle stress in ways that are damaging. They may turn to alcohol, prescription medications, illegal drugs, caffeine, nicotine, or anything they think might lift or calm them. Some choose to binge on food. Any excessive behavior, even gambling or oversleeping, may be a way to try to get away from stress. Few of these solutions work, and with diabetes, most of them are dangerous. There are other, safer stress relievers.

How to Handle Stress Safely

Take a deep breath. Sit or lie down and uncross your legs and arms. Close your eyes. Breathe in deeply and slowly. Let all the

How Do You Handle Stress?

When you are under stress, which of the following do you do? Circle T if the statement is true and F if it is false.

1. Have a few drinks	T	F
2. Talk to a doctor	T	F
3. Have a snack	T	F
4. Call a friend	T	F
5. Smoke	T	F
6. Take a vacation	T	F
7. Ignore my diet	T	F
8. Work on my hobby	T	F
9. Not talk to anyone	T	F
10. Take a walk	T	F

SCORING

- For odd-numbered answers, give yourself 1 point for every F.
- For even-numbered answers, give yourself 1 point for every T.
- If you scored 9 or 10, congratulations. You're skilled at dealing with stress.
- If you scored 7 or 8, you're doing pretty well, but might be falling back on some unhealthy habits or not doing all you can to reduce stress.
- If you scored 6 or less, you could use some tips on dealing with stress (see p. 144–147).

breath out. Breathe in and out again. Start to relax your muscles. Keep breathing in and out. Each time you breathe out, relax your muscles even more. Do this for 5 to 20 minutes. Do it at least once a day.

Let go. Lie down. Close your eyes. Tense, hold, and then release the muscles of each part of your body. Start at your head and work your way down to your feet (see Box on progressive muscle relaxation on p. 148).

Loosen up. Circle, stretch, and shake parts of your body.

Stay active. Some of the best activities for relieving stress are circuit training, cross-country skiing, bicycling, rowing, running, and swimming. If you don't like any of these, find another one you like, and do it often.

Get a massage. Put yourself in the hands of a licensed massage therapist.

Think good thoughts. Your thoughts affect your feelings. Put a rubber band on your wrist. Snap it each time you think a bad thought. Replace that bad thought with a better thought. Or repeat a happy poem, prayer, or quote that calms and focuses you.

Talk about it. Find someone to talk to when something is bothering you. It may make you feel better. Confide in family or friends. Consult a therapist or join a support group. Others may be having the same troubles you are.

Put it on paper. Write down what's bothering you. You may find a solution. Or draw or paint your worries away.

Try something new. Start a hobby or learn a craft. Take a class. Join a club or a team. Volunteer to help others. Form a discussion group on books, movies, or whatever interests you. Start a potluck dinner group.

Get away. Go on a minivacation or overnighter, or take a long weekend. Form a baby-sitting cooperative with other parents so you can get out more.

Listen up. Listen to music you find soothing. Or play a tape of nature sounds, like birds or ocean waves.

Soak in a warm bath. The most comfortable bath water is about the same temperature as your skin. Probably between 85° and 93°F. Linger in the bath for 20 to 30 minutes. Add bubbles or soothing herbs if you like.

Say "no." Especially to things you really don't want to do. You may feel stressed if you take on too much.

Laugh about it. Have a hearty, healthy laugh every day. Seek out funny movies, funny books, and funny people.

Look at nature. Look at the world around you. Flowers, trees, even bugs. The sun, the moon, the stars. Clouds, wind, and rain. Just go outside and spend time there. If you can't go outside, look out a window. Even looking at pictures of trees can help you slow down and relax.

Eat wisely. When you are under stress, your body may use up more B vitamins, vitamin C, protein, and calcium. Replenish your B vitamins by eating more whole grains, nuts, seeds, and beans. Boost your vitamin C with oranges, grapefruits, and broccoli. Beef up your protein with chicken, fish, and egg whites. Stock up your calcium with low-fat milk, yogurt, and cheese.

Sleep on it. Sometimes things look better the next day. Get your 7 to 9 hours of sleep a day.

YOUR SUPPORT NETWORK

There is strength in numbers. You don't have to face the emotions and stresses of diabetes alone. Your family, friends, and mental health professionals can help.

Your Family

Learn as much about diabetes as you can. Then share what you have learned with your family. To help you and your family, there are books, magazines, pamphlets, libraries, classes, support groups, and medical professionals that can explain things.

First, each family member needs to understand what diabetes is, how it is controlled, and how to handle those rare emergencies.

Second, your family will probably need to change some of the foods it eats and when it eats. It is important for everyone to eat well-balanced meals at regular times. Although many people don't want to be on a restricted diet, keep in mind that the meal plan for people with diabetes *is healthy* and not necessarily *restrictive*.

Progressive Muscle Relaxation

1. Close your eyes and breathe slowly and deeply.
2. Start with the muscles in your face, working your way down to your feet and toes.
3. Inhale. Raise your eyebrows. Tense them. Hold for a count of 3. Relax your eyebrows. Exhale.
4. Inhale. Open your mouth and eyes wide. Then close your mouth and eyes tightly. Squeeze. Hold for a count of 3. Relax your eyes and mouth. Exhale.
5. Inhale. Bite down on your teeth. Hold for a count of 3. Relax your jaw. Exhale.
6. Inhale. Pull your shoulders up. Hold for a count of 3. Relax your shoulders. Exhale.
7. Inhale. Tense all the muscles in your arms. Hold for a count of 3. Relax your arms. Exhale.
8. Inhale. Tense all the muscles in your chest and abdomen. Hold for a count of 3. Relax your chest and abdomen. Exhale.
9. Inhale. Tense all the muscles in your legs. Hold for a count of 3. Relax your legs. Exhale.
10. Inhale. Tense all the muscles in your feet. Curl your toes. Hold for a count of 3. Relax your feet. Exhale.
11. Inhale. Exhale any tension that may be lingering in your body. Breathe in energy. Take several more deep, slow breaths. Enjoy the relaxation.
12. Gradually open your eyes.

Third, exercise is just as important as food for good diabetes control. You might bike, swim, or take long walks together. Soon, this new team effort just might add to the quality of life for all family members!

Encourage your mate to be supportive, but not a caretaker; to help you keep to the rules, not break them; to lend a sympathetic ear and share in the process of finding solutions, but not lecture.

Be careful not to shift an unreasonable amount of responsibility for your diabetes care onto your partner. If you do, he or she may resent the time and energy required to help you. Conversely, if you shut your partner out of your diabetes care, he or she may feel a sense of helplessness in not being able to "rescue" you.

It can be frustrating and worrisome for your mate if you don't always eat well, check blood glucose levels, and exercise. Both of you need to realize that no one is perfect! And both of you need to acknowledge that your feelings exist, whatever they are, and to share them honestly.

Your Friends

You decide what to tell friends and how much to tell. Be sure your family knows to follow your guidelines. Just remember that you may, at times, need help.

Tell your friends outright what you need. Help them learn about diabetes by offering to take them along with you to a medical visit or to your diabetes club or support group or by lending them something to read about diabetes. The more your friends know, the better able they will be to help you.

Tell your friends it is okay for them to say no to you when you ask for help. When they do help you, do them a kindness in return, such as shoveling snow, raking leaves, or making dinner.

Your Mental Health Professional

A mental health professional can help you explore your thoughts, feelings, worries, and concerns and look at your inter-actions with others and the decisions you make. Therapy with a mental health professional can help you deal with your emo-tions, discover new approaches to old problems, change your behavior, and learn new ways of coping.

Depending on your needs, you may want individual, couple, family, or group therapy. Group therapy can give you added support and a chance to support others. Sometimes it's easier to find solutions to your problems when you share them and hear about other people's solutions to similar problems.

Find a therapist who supports you. You may need to talk to several before it feels right. See RESOURCES for professional orga-nizations that can make local referrals.

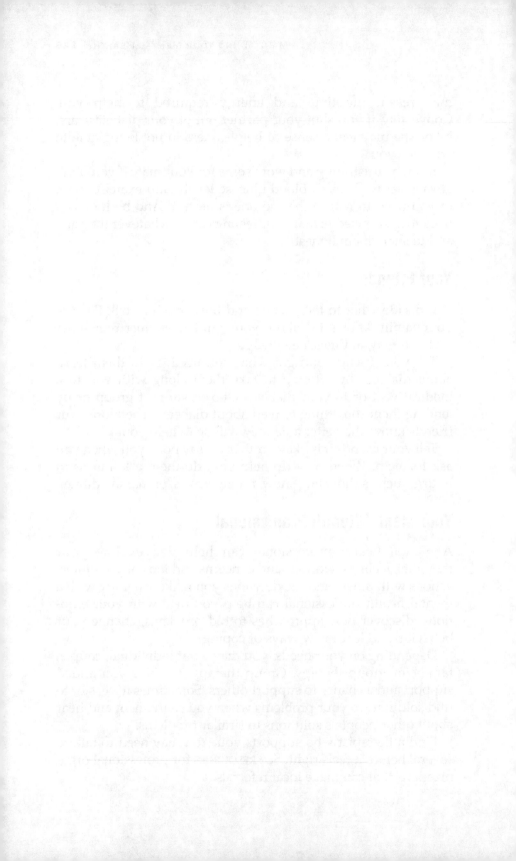

RESOURCES

FOR THE VISUALLY CHALLENGED

American Council of the Blind
1155 15th Street NW, Suite 1004
Washington, DC 20005
202–467–5081
800–424–8666
202–467–5085 (fax)
e-mail: info@acb.org
Web site: http://www.acb.org
National information
clearinghouse and legislative
advocate that publishes a monthly
magazine in Braille, large print,
cassette, and computer disk
versions.

American Foundation for the Blind
11 Penn Plaza, Suite 300
New York, NY 10001
212–502–7600
800–232–5463
e-mail: afbinfo@afb.net

Web site: http://www.afb.org
Works to establish, develop, and
provide services and programs
that assist visually challenged
people in achieving independence.

American Printing House for the Blind
1839 Frankfort Avenue
P.O. Box 6085
Louisville, KY 40206
502–895–2405
502–899–2274 (fax)
800–223–1839
Web site: http://www.aph.org
Concerned with the publication of
literature in all media (Braille,
large type, recorded) and
manufacture of educational aids.
Newsletter provides information
on new products.

National Association for Visually Handicapped (NAVH)
22 West 21st Street
New York, NY 10010
212–889–3141
212–727–2931 (fax)
Web site: http://www.navh.org
or
NAVH San Francisco regional office (for states west of the Mississippi)
3201 Balboa Street
San Francisco, CA 94121
415–221–3201
415–221–8754 (fax)
A list of low-vision facilities is available by state. Visual aid counseling and visual aids, peer support groups, and more intensive counseling are offered at both offices. Some counseling is done by mail or phone. Maintains a large-print loan library.

National Federation of the Blind
1800 Johnson Street
Baltimore, MD 21230
410–659–9314
email: epc@roudley.com
Web site: http://www.nfb.org
Membership organization providing information, networking, and resources through 52 affiliates in all states, the District of Columbia, and Puerto Rico. Some aids and appliances available through national headquarters. The Diabetics Division publishes a free quarterly newsletter, *Voice of the Diabetic*, in print or on cassette.

National Library Service (NLS) for the Blind and Physically Handicapped
Library of Congress
Washington, DC 20542
202–707–5100
202–707–0744 (TDD)
202–707–0712 (fax)
800–424–8567 (to speak with a reference person)
email: nls@loc.gov
Web site: http://www.loc.gov/nls
Publishes *Diabetes Forecast* on cassette. It is available on request through the NLS program to individuals registered with the talking book program.

Recording for the Blind & Dyslexic (RFBD)
20 Roszel Road
Princeton, NJ 08540
609–452–0606
609–987–8116 (fax)
800–803–7201
email: custserv@rfbd.org
Web site: http://www.rfbd.org
Library for people with print disabilities. Provides educational materials in recorded and computerized form; almost 80,000 titles on cassette. Registration fee of $50.00 includes loan of cassettes for up to a year; $25 per year thereafter.

The Seeing Eye, Inc.
P.O. Box 375
Morristown, NJ 07963–0375
973–539–4425
973–539–0922 (fax)
e-mail: semaster@seeingeye.org

Web site: http://www.
seeingeye.org
Offers guide dog training and
instruction on working with a
guide dog.

FOR AMPUTEES

American Amputee Foundation
P.O. Box 250218
Little Rock, AR 72225
501–666–2523
501–666–8367 (fax)
Offers peer counseling for new
amputees and their families.
Provides information and referral
to vendors. Has local chapters.
Maintains a list of support groups
throughout the United States. No
financial assistance offered.

**National Amputation
Foundation**
38–40 Church Street
Malverne, NY 11565
516–887–3600
516–887–3667 (fax)
email: info@nationalamputation.
org
Web site: http://www.
nationalamputation.org
Sponsor of Amp-to-Amp program
in which new amputee is visited
by amputee who has resumed
normal life. A list of support
groups throughout the country is
available.

FOR FINDING LONG-TERM OR HOME CARE

**National Association for Home
Care (NAHC)**
228 7th Street SE
Washington, DC 20003
202–547–7424
202–547–3540 (fax)
email: webmaster@nahc.org
Web site: http://www.nahc.org
Free information for consumers
about how to choose a home care
agency. Searchable online

directory of home care and
hospice agencies.

**Nursing Home Information
Service**
c/o National Council of
Senior Citizens
8403 Colesville Road, Suite 1200
Silver Spring, MD 20910
301–578–8800, ext. 8938
301–578–8999 (fax)

Web site: http://www.nscerc.org/
nursing.htm
Information on selecting and
paying for a nursing home and
choosing other long-term care
alternatives.

FOR FINDING QUALITY HEALTH CARE

**American Association for
Marriage and Family Therapy**
1133 15th Street NW, Suite 300
Washington, DC 20005–2710
202–452–0109
202–223–2329 (fax)
email: central@aamft.org
Web site: http://www.aamft.org
Searchable online directory of
marriage and family therapists.

**American Association of
Diabetes Educators**
100 West Monroe Street, Suite 400
Chicago, IL 60603-1901
312–424–2426
312–424–2427 (fax)
800–832–6874
email: aade@aadenet.org
Web site: http://www.aadenet.
org
Referral to a local diabetes
educator. Searchable online
directory of diabetes educators.

**American Association of Sex
Educators, Counselors, and
Therapists**
P.O. Box 238
Mount Vernon, IA 52314–0238
319–895–6203 (fax)
email: aasect@worldnet.att.net
Web site: http://www.aasect.org

For a list of certified sex therapists
and counselors in any state, send
request along with a self-
addressed, stamped, business-size
envelope. Searchable online
directory of certified sex
therapists and counselors.

**American Board of Medical
Specialties**
1007 Church Street, Suite 404
Evanston, IL 60201—5913
847–491–9091
847–328–3596 (fax)
800–776–2378
Web site:http://www.certified
doctor.org
Record of physicians certified by
24 medical specialty boards. Only
certification status of physician is
available to callers. Directories of
certified physicians organized by
city of medical practice and
alphabetically by physician
names are available in many
libraries. Searchable online
directory of certified physicians.

**American Board of Podiatric
Surgery**
3330 Mission Street
San Francisco, CA 94110–5009
415–826–3200

415–826–4640 (fax)
email: info@abps.org
Web site: http://www.abps.org
Referral to a local board-certified
podiatrist.

The American Dietetic Association
216 West Jackson Boulevard
Chicago, IL 60606–6995
312–899–0040
312–899–1979 (fax)
800–366–1655 Consumer
    Nutrition Hot Line; 9–4 CST,
    M–F only
Web site: http://www.
    eatright.org
Information, guidance, and
referral to a local dietitian.

American Medical Association
515 North State Street
Chicago, IL 60610
312–464–5000
Web site: http://www.
    ama–assn.org
Referral to your county or state
medical society, which may be
able to refer you to a local
physician.

American Optometric Association
243 N. Lindbergh Boulevard
St. Louis, MO 63141
314–991–4100
314–991–4101 (fax)
Web site: http://www.
    aoanet.org/
Referral to your state optometric
association for referral to a local
optometrist.

American Psychiatric Association
1400 K Street NW
Washington, DC 20005
202–682–6000
202–682–6850 (fax)
888–357–7924
Web site: http://www.psych.org
Referral to your state psychiatric
association for referral to a local
psychiatrist.

American Psychological Association
750 First Street NE
Washington, DC 20002–4242
202–336–5500 (main number)
202–336–5700 (public affairs)
202–436–5800 (professional
    practice)
800–374–2721
Web site: http://www.apa.org
Referral to your state
psychological association for
referral to a local psychologist.

National Association of Social Workers
750 First Street NE, Suite 700
Washington, DC 20002–4247
202–408–8600
800–638–8799
email: info@naswdc.org
Web site: http://naswdc.org
Referral to your state chapter of
NASW for referral to a local social
worker.

Pedorthic Footwear Association
9861 Broken Land Parkway,
Suite 255
Columbia, MD 21046–1151
410–381–7278
410–381–1167 (fax)
800–673–8447

email: info@pfa.org
Referral to a local certified
pedorthist (a person trained in
fitting prescription footwear).
Searchable online directory of
pedorthists.

FOR MISCELLANEOUS HEALTH INFORMATION

**American Academy of
Ophthalmology**
Customer Service Department
655 Beach Street
San Francisco, CA 94109–1336
415–561–8500
415–561–8575 (fax)
email: comm@aao.org
Web site: http://www.eyenet.org
For brochures on eye care and eye
diseases, send a self-addressed,
stamped envelope. Searchable
online directory of
opthalmologists.

American Heart Association
7272 Greenville Avenue
Dallas, TX 75231
800–242–8721
Web site: http://www.amhrt.org
For referral to local affiliate's
Heartline, which provides
information on cardiovascular
health and disease prevention.

Impotence World Association
119 S. Ruth Street
Maryville, TN 37803
800–669–1603
email: iwatenn@aol.com

For information and guidance on
impotence and physician referral
in your state, send a written
request; a stamped, self-
addressed envelope; and $2.00.

Medic Alert Foundation
P.O. Box 819008
Turlock, CA 95381–1009
209–668–3333
209–669–2450 (fax)
800–432–5378
e-mail: customer_service@
   medicalert.org
Web site: http://www.medicalert.
   org

National AIDS Hot Line
Centers for Disease Control and
   Prevention
800–342–2437 (24 hours)
800–344–7432 (Spanish)
800–243–7889 (TTY)
Information on HIV and AIDS,
including pamphlets and
brochures, counseling, and
referral to local test sites, case
managers, and medical services.

National Chronic Pain Outreach Association
7979 Old Georgetown Road, Suite 100
Bethesda, MD 20814–2429
301–652–4948
301–907–0745 (fax)
To learn more about chronic pain and how to deal with it.

National Kidney Foundation
30 E. 33rd Street, Suite 1100
New York, NY 10016
212–889–2210
212–689–9261 (fax)
800–622–9010
e-mail: info@kidney.org

Web site: http://www.kidney.org
For donor cards and information about kidney disease and transplants.

United Network for Organ Sharing
1100 Boulders Parkway, Suite 500
P.O. Box 13770
Richmond, VA 23225–8770
800–894–6361 (for information on becoming a donor)
800–24–DONOR
For information about organ transplants and a list of organ transplant centers in the U.S.

FOR TRAVELERS

U.S. Government Printing Office
Superintendent of Documents
P.O. Box 371954
Pittsburgh, PA 15250–7954
202–512–1800
202–512–2250 (fax)
Order the brochure *Health Information for International Travelers* (stock # 017–023–001957) by phone with credit card or send check or money order for $14.

International Association for Medical Assistance to Travelers
417 Center Street
Lewiston, NY 14092
716–754–4883

For a list of doctors in foreign countries who speak English and who received postgraduate training in North America or Great Britain.

International Diabetes Federation
40 Washington Street
B–1050 Brussels, Belgium
Web site: http://www.idf.org
For a list of International Diabetes Federation groups that can offer assistance when you're traveling.

FOR EXERCISERS

American College of Sports Medicine
P.O. Box 1440
Indianapolis, IN 46206–1440
317–637–9200
317–634–7817 (fax)
e-mail: astrobec@ascm.org
Web site: http://www.acsm.org
For information about health and fitness.

International Diabetic Athletes Association
1647 W. Bethany Home Road, #B
Phoenix, AZ 85015–2507
800–898–4322
e-mail: idaa@diabetes–exercise.org

Web site: http://www.getnet.com/~idaa/
For people with diabetes and for health care professionals interested in exercise and fitness at all levels. Newsletter.

President's Council on Physical Fitness and Sports
200 Independence Avenue, SW
Humphrey Building, Room 738H
Washington, DC 20201
202–690–9000
202–690–5211 (fax)
For information about physical activity, exercise, and fitness.

FOR PEOPLE OVER 50

American Association of Retired Persons (AARP)
601 E Street NW
Washington, DC 20049
202–434–2277
202–434–2558 (fax)
Web site: http://www.aarp.org
800–424–3410 (membership)
800–456–2277 (mail-order pharmacy)
Over-the-counter and prescription drugs delivered to your door in 7 to 10 days. Competitive prices that are the same for members and nonmembers. May pay by credit card or be billed.

National Council on the Aging
409 3rd Street SW
2nd Floor
Washington, DC 20024
202–479–1200
202–479–0735 (fax)
e-mail: info@ncoa.org
Web site: http://www.ncoa.org
Advocacy group concerned with developing and implementing high standards of care for the elderly. Referral to local agencies concerned with the elderly.

FOR EQUAL EMPLOYMENT INFORMATION

American Bar Association
Commission on Mental and
  Physical Disability Law
740 15th Street NW
Washington, DC 20005–1009
202–662–1570
202–662–1032 (fax)
202–662–1012 (TTY)
Web site: http://www.abanet.org/
  disability
Provides information and
technical assistance on all aspects
of disability law.

**Disability Rights Education and
Defense Fund, Inc.**
2212 6th Street
Berkeley, CA 94710
510–644–2555 (voice/TTY)
510–841–8645 (fax)
e-mail: dredf@dredf.org
Provides technical assistance and
information to employers and
individuals with disabilities on
disability rights legislation and
policies. Assists with legal
representation.

**Equal Employment Opportunity
Commission**
1801 L Street NW
Washington, DC 20507
For technical assistance and filing
  a charge:
202–663–4900
202–663–4912 (fax)
800–669–4000 (connects to nearest
  local EEOC office)
800–669–3362 (for publications)
800–800–3302 (TDD)

**National Information Center for
Children and Youth With
Disabilities**
P.O. Box 1492
Washington, DC 20013–1492
202–884–8200 (voice and TTY)
202–884–8441 (fax)
800–695–0285 (voice and TTY)
e-mail: nichcy@aed.org
Web site: http://www.nichcy.org
Provides technical assistance and
information on disabilities and
disability-related issues.

FOR HEALTH INSURANCE INFORMATION

AARP health insurance
800–523–5800
The AARP administers 10 health
insurance plans. For some plans,
individuals with diabetes or other
chronic illnesses are eligible
within 6 months after enrolling in

Medicare Part B. For other plans,
a 3-month waiting period is
required for those with conditions
preexistent in the 6 months
preceding the effective date of the
insurance, if not replacing
previous coverage.

Medicare Hot Line
800–638–6833
U.S. Department of Health and
 Human Services
Health Care Financing
 Administration
6325 Security Boulevard
Baltimore, MD 21207

For information and various
publications about Medicare.

Social Security Administration
800–772–1213
For information and various
publications about Medicare.

AMERICAN DIABETES ASSOCIATION REGIONAL OFFICES

Great Lakes/Heartland Region
2323 North Mayfair Road, #502
Wauwatosa, WI 53226
414/778-5500

South Coastal Region
1101 North Lake Destiny Road,
 Suite 415
Maitland, FL 32751
407/660-1926

Western Region
10445 Old Placerville Road
Sacramento, CA 95827
916/369-0999

Mid-Atlantic Region
8300 Professional Place, Suite 105
Landover, MD 20785
240/737-2000

Eastern/New England Region
7 Washington Square
Albany, NY 12205
518/218-1755

South Central Region
4425 West Airport Freeway,
 Suite 130
Irving, TX 75062
972/255-6900

Southern Region
2 Hanover Square, Suite 1600
434 Fayetteville Street Mall
Raleigh, NC 27601
919/743-5400

Mid-America Region
P.O. Box 1013
Columbia, MO 65205
573/443-8611

**Mountain States/Pacific NW
Region**
2450 South Downing Street
Denver, CO 80210
720/855-1102

INDEX

Acarbose, 77–78
Age, risk factor for diabetes, 3, 6
AIDS, 156
Albumin, 109
Alcohol
  calories, 131, 132
  complications and, 113
  cooking with, 133
  driving and, 131
  exchanges, 132
  low blood glucose and, 130–131
  meal plan, including in, 131
  pregnancy and, 74
Alpha-glucosidase inhibitors, 77–78
American Association of Diabetes
  Educators, 20, 154
American Diabetes Association Regional
  Offices, 160
American Dietetic Association, The,
  16–17, 155
Americans With Disabilities Act of 1990,
  121–122
Amputation, 67, 105, 153
Anger, 137–138
Angina, 103
Arterial bypass surgery, 104, 105
Assertiveness, 142
Atherectomy, 104, 105
Atherosclerosis, 103, 104
Athlete's foot, 64
Autonomic neuropathy, 112–114

Balloon angioplasty, 103–104, 105
Biguanides, 77
Blood fats (lipids), 115–116

Blood glucose
  effect of medications on, 80–81
  high, 97–98, 102
  low, 94–97
  meters, 92–94
  record-keeping, 91–92
  self-monitoring of. *See* Self-monitoring
    of blood glucose
Blood lipids (fats), 115–116
Blood pressure, 99, 100, 102, 114–115. *See*
  also High blood pressure
Blood testing
  cholesterol, 115–116
  glycohemoglobin, 100
  triglycerides, 115–116
Blood vessels, 102, 105, 113
Body fat
  distribution, 3
  insulin resistance, 3
Body mass index, 5
Body weight, 4
Boils, 64
Brain, 104–105, 113
Breast-feeding, 74

Caffeine, 133
Calluses, 66
Carbohydrate, 38–39
Carbohydrate counting, 49–50
Carbuncle, 64
Cardiovascular disease. *See* Heart
  disease
Carotid endarterectomy, 105
Carpal tunnel syndrome, 114
Cataracts, 108

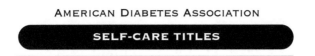
American Diabetes Association Complete Guide to Diabetes, 2nd Edition

Every area of self-care is covered in this ultimate diabetes reference for your home. With it, you can solve problems with hundreds of hints, tips, and tricks that are proven to work. It covers insulin use. Blood sugar control. Sex and pregnancy. Eating and weight control. Insurance. Mastering diabetes supplies. Every aspect of your daily and professional life. You'll turn to this all-in-one guide again and again!
Softcover. #4809-02 Nonmember: $23.95/ADA Member: $19.95

NEW!

The Uncomplicated Guide to Diabetes Complications

Thorough, comprehensive chapters cover everything you need to know about preventing and treating diabetes complications in simple language that everyone can understand. Covers kidney disease, heart disease, obesity, eye disease, sexual disorders, hypertension and stroke, neuropathy and vascular disease, and more.
Softcover. #4814-01
Nonmember: $18.95 Member: $16.95

101 Tips for Staying Healthy with Diabetes, 2nd Edition

Get the inside track on the latest tips, techniques, and strategies for preventing and treating diabetes complications. You'll learn how to treat and prevent skin infections, which cold and flu medicines to avoid, and how to eat the foods you like healthful.
Softcover. #4810-01
$14.95

12 Things You Must Know About Diabetes Care Right Now!

This book explains the ADA Standards of Care and informs you of the importance of seeking medical attention that meets these standards. Includes discussions on the different types of diabetes, the goals of treatment, how to choose and effectively talk to your doctor, and more.
Softcover. #4811-02
$14.95

NEW!

The American Diabetes Association Guide to Healthy Restaurant Eating

What to Eat in America's Most Popular Family and Chain Restaurants

Introducing your complete guide to what's in when you're in the mood to eat out. You'll instantly have access to complete nutrition information for selections at Arby's, Burger King, Wendy's, McDonald's, Boston Market, Kentucky Fried Chicken, Popeye's, Long John Silver's, and dozens of others. Plus, you no longer have to avoid sugary foods and sweets, so you can enjoy your favorite treats at Baskin Robbins, TCBY, and many more! You'll learn just how healthy and enjoyable eating out can be, even with diabetes.

Softcover. #4819-01
Nonmember: $13.95 Member: $11.95

NEW!

The Commonsense Guide to Weight Loss for People with Diabetes

This book dispels the myths about dieting and shows you how to lose weight—and keep it off—using commonsense techniques. You'll learn seven crucial elements of weight loss for people with diabetes:

• Choosing the right target weight
• Measuring weight-loss progress by tracking health, not weight
• Developing a healthy, low-calorie diet while enjoying tasty, filling meals
• Coordinating a weight-loss program with proper diabetes care
• Improving your weight-loss program with modern medicine
• Maintaining an active lifestyle
• Making permanent lifestyle changes to ensure long-term weight loss

Softcover. #4816-01
Nonmemnber: $19.95 Member: $17.95

101 Tips for Improving Your Blood Sugar, 2nd Edition

101 Tips offers a practical, easy-to-follow road map to tight blood sugar control. One question appears on each page, with the answers or "tips" below each question. Tips on diet, exercise, travel, weight loss, insulin, illness, and more.

Softcover. #4805-01
$14.95

Diabetes A to Z, 4th Edition

In clear, simple terms, you'll learn all about blood glucose, complications, diet, exercise, heart disease, insulin, kidney disease, meal planning, pregnancy, sex, weight loss, and much more. Alphabetized for quick reference.
Softcover. #4801-04
$14.95

Managing Diabetes on a Budget

For less than $10 you can begin saving hundreds and hundreds on your diabetes self-care. An inexpensive, sure-fire collection of tips and hints to save you money on everything from medications and diet to exercise and health care.
Softcover. #5002-01
Nonmember: $7.95/Member: $6.95

The Uncomplicated Guide to Diabetes Complications

A comprehensive and concise guide to diabetes complications—what they are, what they mean, and what treatments are available. Learn everything you need to know about preventing, treating, and caring for complications like heart and kidney disease, hypertension and stroke, neuropathy and vascular disease, and others.
Softcover. #4814-01
Nonmember: $18.95 Member: $16.95

Caring for the Diabetic Soul

This book will help you deal with the emotional challenges of diabetes care—the thoughts, feelings, and fears that must be faced every day. You'll learn about:
• Coping with denial
• Controlling your stress and anger
• Building self-esteem
• Much more
Softcover. #4815-01
Nonmember $9.95 Member $8.95

Meditations on Diabetes: Strengthening Your Spirit in Every Season

You will be encouraged by meditations from • Jesse Jackson • Mother Teresa • Mark Twain • Eleanor Roosevelt • Albert Einstein • and many more in this book that will help heal and strengthen your spirit by starting at the root of it all—your soul.
Softcover. #4820-01
Nonmember: $13.95 Member: $11.95

The American Diabetes Association 2000 Resource Guide

#5512-01
$3.95

101 Foot Care Tips for People with Diabetes

Helpful treatment advice and do's and don'ts of foot care. Leading physicians discuss the best shoes to wear, how to get a good fit, what to do if you find a cut, how to avoid foot ulcers, and more.
Softcover. #4834-01
$14.95

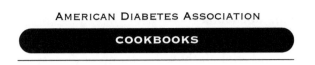

How to Cook for People with Diabetes

Finally, a collection of reader favorites from the delicious, nutritious recipes featured every month in *Diabetes Forecast*. But you don't only get ideas for pizza, chicken, unique holiday foods, vegetarian recipes and more, you also get nutrient analysis and exchanges for each recipe.
Softcover. #4616-01
Nonmember: $11.95/ADA Member: $9.95

World-Class Diabetic Cooking

Travel around the world at every meal with a collection of 200 exciting new low-fat, low-calorie recipes. Features recipes from Thailand, Italy, Greece, Spain, China, Japan, Africa, Mexico, Germany, and more. Appetizers, soups, salads, pastas, meats, breads, and desserts are highlighted.
Softcover. #4617-01
Nonmember: $12.95/Member: $10.95

Southern-Style Diabetic Cooking

This cookbook takes traditional Southern dishes and turns them into great-tasting recipes you'll come back to again and again. Features more than 100 recipes including appetizers, main dishes, and desserts; complete nutrient analysis with each recipe, and suggestions for modifying recipes to meet individual nutritional needs.
Softcover. #4615-01
Nonmember: $11.95/Member: $9.95

Flavorful Seasons Cookbook

Warm up your winter with recipes for Christmas, welcome spring with an Easter recipe, and cool off those hot summer days with more recipes for the Fourth of July. More than 400 unforgettable choices that combine great taste with all the good-for-you benefits of a well-balanced meal. Cornish Game Hens, Orange Sea Bass, Ginger Bread Pudding, many others.
Softcover. #4613-01
Nonmember: $16.95/Member: $14.95

Diabetic Meals In 30 Minutes—Or Less!

Put an end to bland, time-consuming meals with more than 140 fast, flavorful recipes. Complete nutrition information accompanies every recipe. A number of "quick tips" will have you out of the kitchen and into the dining room even faster! Salsa Salad, Oven-Baked Parmesan Zucchini, Roasted Red Pepper Soup, Layered Vanilla Parfait, and more.
Softcover. #4614-01
Nonmember: $11.95/Member: $9.95

Diabetes Meal Planning Made Easy, 2nd Edition

Learn quick and easy ways to eat more starches, fruits, vegetables, and milk; make changes in your eating habits to reach your goals; and understand how to use the Nutrition Facts on food labels. You'll also master the intricacies of each food group in the new Diabetes Food Pyramid.
Softcover. #4706-02
$14.95

Month of Meals: Classic Cooking

When celebrations begin, go ahead—dig in! Includes a Special Occasion section that offers tips for brunches, holidays, and restaurants to give you delicious dining options anytime, anywhere. Menu choices include Chicken Cacciatore, Oven-Fried Fish, Sloppy Joes, Crab Cakes, and many others.
Softcover. #4701-01
$14.95

Month of Meals: Ethnic Delights

Automatic menu planning goes ethnic! Tips and meal suggestions for Mexican, Italian, and Chinese restaurants are featured. Quick-to-fix and ethnic recipes are also included. Beef Burritos, Chop Suey, Veal Piccata, Stuffed Peppers, and others.
Softcover. #4702-01 $14.95

Month of Meals: Meals in Minutes

Enjoy fast food without guilt! Make delicious choices at McDonald's, Wendy's, Taco Bell, and other fast-food restaurants. Special sections offer valuable tips, such as reading ingredient labels, preparing meals for picnics, and meal planning when you're ill.
Softcover. #4703-01 $14.95

Month of Meals: Old-Time Favorites

Meat and potatoes menu planning! Enjoy old-time family favorites like Meatloaf and Pot Roast, Crispy Fried Chicken, Beef Stroganoff, and many others. Hints for turning family-size meals into delicious leftovers will keep generous portions from going to waste. Meal plans for one or two people are also featured. Spiral-bound.
Softcover. #4704-01 $14.95

Month of Meals: Vegetarian Pleasures

Meatless meals picked fresh from the garden. Choose from a garden of fresh vegetarian selections like Eggplant Italian, Stuffed Zucchini, Cucumbers with Dill Dressing, Vegetable Lasagna, and many others. Plus, you'll reap all the health benefits of a vegetarian diet.
Softcover. #4705-01 $14.95

Cooking with the Diabetic Chef

Written for people with diabetes by a chef with diabetes—150 recipes that satisfy your cravings. You can eat the foods you love and live healthy with diabetes. Recipes include chocolate chip pancakes, steak teriyaki, melt-in-your-mouth ribs. Best of all, they're easy to prepare.
Softcover. #4630-01
$19.95

Quick & Easy Diabetic Recipes for One

Cook for one without wasting food, tossing out leftovers, or cutting recipes in half and in half again. 100 recipes, plus tips on shopping, preparation and more.
Softcover. #4621-01
Nonmember: $12.95 Member: $10.95

The Great Chicken Cookbook

Chicken any way you want it but always tasty, always healthy. The 150 low-fat recipes cover a wide variety of ethnic traditions, giving you dishes that explode with flavor. Try Chicken Shish Kabob, Chicken Morengo, and Deviled Chicken Legs.
Softcover. #4627-01
Nonmember: $16.95 Member: $14.95

The NEW Family Cookbook for People with Diabetes

Even the most finicky eaters love these tasty recipes—all 375 of them. Serve Cheddar Cheese Dip, Spicy Chicken Thighs, Mushroom Risotto, and New York Cheesecake without guilt because every recipe adheres to ADA recommendations.
Hardcover. #4618-01
$30.00

HOW TO ORDER

1. **To order by phone**: just call us at **1-800-ADA-ORDER (232-6733)** and have your credit card ready. VISA, MasterCard, and American Express are accepted. Please mention code CK497T2 when ordering.

2. **To order by mail:** on a separate sheet of paper, write down the books you're ordering and calculate the total using the shipping & handling chart below. (NOTE: Virginia residents add 4.5% sales tax; Georgia residents add 7% sales tax.) Then include your check, written to the American Diabetes Association, with your order and mail to:

> **American Diabetes Association**
> Order Fulfillment Department
> P.O. Box 930850
> Atlanta, GA 31193-0850

Shipping & Handling Chart

up to $25.00 ....add $4.99
$25.01-$60.00 ....add $5.99
over $60.00 ....add 10%

Allow 2–3 weeks for shipment. Add $4.00 to shipping & handling for each extra shipping address. Add $15 for each overseas shipment. Prices subject to change without notice.

NOW HERE'S A RECIPE FOR SUCCESSFUL DIABETES SELF-CARE

Yes, I want to join the American Diabetes Association. I've enclosed $28 annual dues.* I will receive 12 issues of *Diabetes Forecast*, membership in my local affiliate, and discounts on all ADA publications.

Name _____

Address _____

_____

City _____ State _____ Zip _____

Telephone _____

Please mail this form with payment to:

American Diabetes Association
General Membership
P.O. Box 363
Mt. Morris, IL 61054-0363

ABK197

*75% of dues is designated for your *Diabetes Forecast* subscription. Allow 6–8 weeks for your first issue of *Diabetes Forecast*. Foreign dues $59. Canadian dues $46 (GST included). Mexican dues $43. All dues must be paid in U.S. funds drawn on a U.S. bank. The IRS requires that we inform you that dues are not deductible for Federal income tax purposes.

About the American Diabetes Association

The American Diabetes Association is the nation's leading voluntary health organization supporting diabetes research, information, and advocacy. Its mission is to prevent and cure diabetes and to improve the lives of all people affected by diabetes. The American Diabetes Association is the leading publisher of comprehensive diabetes information. Its huge library of practical and authoritative books for people with diabetes covers every aspect of self-care—cooking and nutrition, fitness, weight control, medications, complications, emotional issues, and general self-care.

To order American Diabetes Association books: Call 1-800-232-6733. http://store.diabetes.org [Note: there is no need to use **www** when typing this particular Web address]

To join the American Diabetes Association: Call 1-800-806-7801. www.diabetes.org/membership

For more information about diabetes or ADA programs and services: Call 1-800-342-2383. E-mail: Customerservice@diabetes.org www.diabetes.org

To locate an ADA/NCQA Recognized Provider of quality diabetes care in your area: Call 1-703-549-1500 ext. 2202. www.diabetes.org/recognition/Physicians/ListAll.asp

To find an ADA Recognized Education Program in your area: Call 1-888-232-0822. www.diabetes.org/recognition/education.asp

To join the fight to increase funding for diabetes research, end discrimination, and improve insurance coverage: Call 1-800-342-2383. www.diabetes.org/advocacy

To find out how you can get involved with the programs in your community: Call 1-800-342-2383. See below for program Web addresses.

- *American Diabetes Month:* Educational activities aimed at those diagnosed with diabetes— month of November. www.diabetes.org/ADM
- *American Diabetes Alert:* Annual public awareness campaign to find the undiagnosed—held the fourth Tuesday in March. www.diabetes.org/alert
- *The Diabetes Assistance & Resources Program (DAR):* diabetes awareness program targeted to the Latino community. www.diabetes.org/DAR
- *African American Program:* diabetes awareness program targeted to the African American community. www.diabetes.org/africanamerican
- *Awakening the Spirit: Pathways to Diabetes Prevention & Control:* diabetes awareness program targeted to the Native American community. www.diabetes.org/awakening

To find out about an important research project regarding type 2 diabetes: www.diabetes.org/ada/research.asp

To obtain information on making a planned gift or charitable bequest: Call 1-888-700-7029. www.diabetes.org/ada/plan.asp

To make a donation or memorial contribution: Call 1-800-342-2383. www.diabetes.org/ada/cont.asp